Stroke: Therapy and Rehabilitation

Other titles published in association with *Hospital Medicine* and the *International Journal of Therapy and Rehabilitation*:

Current Reviews of Otorhinolaryngology, Head and Neck edited by Andrew Swift

Tools for Continuing Professional Development edited by Chia Swee Hong and Deborah Harrison

Stroke: Therapy and Rehabilitation

edited by
Richard White

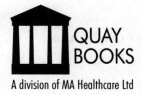

QUAY
BOOKS

A division of MA Healthcare Ltd

Quay Books Division, MA Healthcare Ltd, St Jude's Church, Dulwich Road, London SE24 0PB

British Library Cataloguing-in-Publication Data
A catalogue record is available for this book

© MA Healthcare Limited 2005
ISBN 1 85642 247 X

Printed in the UK by Ashford Colour Press Ltd, Gosport, Hants

CONTENTS

LIST OF CONTRIBUTORS

Ruth Baker is Head of Physiotherapy, Haringey Primary Care Trust, St Anne's Hopsital, London

Holly Blake is Research Psychologist, University of Nottingham, Nottingham

Sharon Burrows is Clinical Development Facilitator, Tower Hamlets Primary Care Trust, Mile End Hospital, London

M Anne Chamberlain is Charterhouse Professor of Rehabilitation Medicine, School of Medicine, University of Leeds

Philippa Clark is Stroke Services Coordinator, Tower Hamlets Primary Care Trust, Mile End Hospital, London

Lynn K Dangerfield is Specialist Speech and Language Therapist, Stroke Service, Queen Alexandra Hospital, Portsmouth

George Dowswell is Senior Research Fellow, Department of Applied Social Science, University of Manchester, Manchester

Therese Dowswell is Senior Research Fellow, Faculty of Medicine, Dentistry, Psychology and Health, University of Leeds

Judi Edmans is Senior Occupational Therapist, Nottingham City Hospital, Nottingham

Angela Gall is Specialist Registrar, Department of Rehabilitation Medicine, Woodend Hospital, Aberdeen, Scotland

Joanna Geddes is Senior Research Fellow, School of Medicine, University of Leeds, Leeds

Patrick Gompertz is Consultant Physician, Queen Mary's School Medicine and Dentistry, Royal London Hospital, London

John Green is Research Physiotherapist, St Luke's Hospital, Bradford

Jane Greene is Stroke Nurse Specialist, ADPC Office, Edenderry House, Portadown, Ireland

Tammy Hoffmann is Associate Lecturer, Division of Occupational Therapy, School of Health and Rehabilitation Sciences, University of Queensland, Queensland, Australia

Terri Horton is Head of Adult Speech and Language Therapy Department, Thames Gateway NHS Trust, Medway Maritime Hospital, Gillingham, Kent

Penny Irwin is Programme Coordinator for Stroke, Royal College of Physicians, London, UK

John Lawler is Lecturer in Leadership and Management, Nuffield Institute for Health, University of Leeds, Leeds

Nadina B Lincoln is Professor of Clinical Psychology, School of Psychology, University of Nottingham, Nottingham

Kryss McKenna is Senior Lecturer, Division of Occupational Therapy, School of Health and Rehabilitation Sciences, University of Queensland, Queensland, Australia

Christopher McKevitt is Research Fellow in Social Sciences, Guy's, King's and St Thomas's Hospital Medical School, London

Joan Murphy is Research Speech and Language Therapist, Department of Psychology, University of Stirling, Stirling, Scotland

Jo Pethybridge is Team Leader, Campden Primary Care Trust, London, UK; her colleague, Yvonne Webb, is also based in London

Majnu Pushpangadan is Specialist Registrar in General Medicine/Medicine for the Elderly, Leeds General Infirmary, Leeds

Deborah JC Ramsey is Research Fellow in Stroke Medicine, William Harvey Hospital, Kent

Stephen J Read is Coordinator of Stroke Services, Department of Neurology, Royal Brisbane Hospital, Australia

Anthony Rudd is Consultant Physician for Stroke, St Thomas' Hospital, London

Andrew Slack is Senior House Officer, Department of Renal Medicine, Guy's and St Thomas's Trust, London

David G Smithard is Consultant in Elderly and Stroke Medicine, William Harvey Hospital, Kent

Ruth A Sullivan is Speech and Language Therapist, Lead Practitioner, Adult Services, South Weald and Downs Community Trust, Chichester

Mira Vogel is Research Fellow, Department of Health for Older People, Queen Mary's School Medicine and Dentistry, Royal London Hospital, London

Charles Wolfe is Reader in Public Health Sciences, Guy's, King's and St Thomas's Hospital Medical School, London

Linda Worrall is Associate Professor, Division of Speech Pathology, School of Health and Rehabilitation Sciences, University of Queensland, Queensland, Australia

John Wright is Consultant in Epidemiology and Public Health, Bradford Royal Infirmary, West Yorkshire

John Young is Professor and Consultant Geriatrician, St Luke's Hospital, Bradford, West Yorkshire

FOREWORD

This book contains a collection of chapters derived from recently reported primary research based papers that have been published in a variety of healthcare journals. That the papers originally appeared in such a wide range of medical and nursing journals is testimony to the complex nature of stroke and the need to have multiprofessional healthcare teams managing and caring for the patient. Stroke management places a requirement on all healthcare professionals to have an understanding of the care and management of this client group and the ability to work seamlessly in an interprofessional approach, respecting and valuing the unique contribution that each team player brings to the clinical setting.

Some 130,000 people in England and Wales will have a stroke each year and there are more than 250,000 people living with the after-effects of stroke, absorbing some 4% of the NHS budget and making stroke the largest cause of disability. This level of incidence and prevalence is common to most developed societies.

Providing the best care — ie. care that is effective and efficient for patients — is central to healthcare professionals' thinking and is their *raison d'être*; yet that is not always easy to do in practice. Conflicting approaches and a plethora of sources of information leave the clinician, be that doctor, nurse or therapist, with a bewildering volume of data on which to base clinical decisions. The development of the *National Clinical Guidelines for Stroke* by the Intercollegiate Working Party for Stroke, a multidisciplinary group representing all the Royal Colleges together with service-user and carer groups, provides a comprehensive guide on the best care pathways for stroke patients (Royal College of Physicians [RCP], 2004a). This book brings together much of the evidence that led to the development of the guidelines and is presented in the form of a patient journey.

The book covers acute stroke management, stroke rehabilitation in both hospital and community settings, as well management of specific commonly found problems such as dysphagia, communication, cognitive impairments, affective impairments and management of the hemiplegic arm. In addition to clinical issues, the chapters also cover service development such as stroke units, evidence-based guidelines and the *National Clinical Guidelines for Stroke*. In this sense, the text has something for everyone.

This collection provides evidence that appropriate care and management of the stroke patient can bring about huge differences in the outcomes for those who suffer a stroke in terms of their survival and quality of life. Those concerned with caring for stroke patients can develop their knowledge and skills in this area, and be proud of the service they offer.

Bernard Gibbon
Head of Department of Nursing
University of Central Lancashire
August 2005

INTRODUCTION

Someone in the UK has a stroke every five minutes and 48% are dead or disabled at six months (Mant, 2004; cited by Rodgers and Rudd, 2004). This puts the clinical reality of stroke in a clear light.

The idea for this book came following a spate of excellent articles on stroke and rehabilitation in the *British Journal of Therapy and Rehabilitation* (*BJTR*). This is not my general reading (my interests lie in dermatology and wound management), but everyone has a relative or friend who has suffered a stroke, so everyone has an interest. What struck me about these articles was the focus of the authors — there was a clear pathway to stroke rehabilitation, and it had been published. This led me to look further afield. I tend to regard SIGN guidelines as the pinnacle of what we in health care should follow. Sure enough, SIGN had provided guideline 64, 'The management of patients with stroke part IV: Rehabilitation, prevention and management of complications, and discharge planning'. There is evidence in this document that deserves quotation:

In comparison with a general hospital ward, the benefits of stroke rehabilitation in an organised hospital stroke unit provides:

> *18% reduction in death*
> *20% reduction in death or institutional care*
> *2% reduction in death or dependency.*

All are statistically significant.

However, according to the *National Service Framework for Older People*, every hospital treating stroke patients was supposed to have a specialist unit in operation by April 2004 and so provide stroke unit care; this has not yet fully materialised (Irwin, Hoffman *et al*, 2005).

Given the facilities, and the resources, high-quality stroke care can be routinely provided. The following chapters are testimony to the rehabilitation available.

Dr Richard White
Whitstone, UK, 2005

References

Irwin P, Hoffman A, Lowe D, Pearson M, Rudd AG (2005) Improving clinical practice in stroke through audit: results of three rounds of National Stroke Audit. *J Eval Clin Pract* **11**: 306–14

Mant J, Wade D, Winner S (2004) Health care needs assessment: stroke. In: Stevens A, Raftery J, Mant J, Simpson S (eds) *Heath Care Needs Assessment: the Epidemiologically Based Needs Assessment Reviews*. 2nd Edition. Radcliffe Medical Press, Oxford

Rodgers H, Rudd A (2004) Quality of stroke care in 2004. *Hosp Med* **65**(9): 519

CHAPTER 1

Management of stroke: acute, rehabilitation and long-term care

David G Smithard

Stroke is the major cause of disability in adults, resulting in much morbidity and mortality in the west. Each year, 120,000 people will suffer their first stroke with a further 40,000 suffering a recurrent stroke and 40,000 a transient ischaemic attack. The prevalence rises from 2/1000 population to 2/100 in those over 85 years of age. Consequently, stroke is seen as a problem of the elderly.

During the acute phase and post-acute phases of stroke, clinical management is often, at best, haphazard. This has been borne out by the National Sentinel Audit of Stroke (Rudd *et al*, 1999), which has revealed that although 75% of trusts have a stroke unit, only about 25% of patients actually spend a significant amount of time in them.

Following the first two National Sentinel Audits of Stroke (Rudd *et al*, 1999; Intercollegiate Working Party for Stroke, 2001) detailing the deficits in provision of stroke care in the UK, the Government included the care of stroke patients (standard 5) in the *National Service Framework (NSF) for Older People* (Department of Health [DoH], 2001). Despite this, the standards pertain to all stroke patients irrespective of age (*Table 1.1*). The NSF contains a timeframe against which stroke services need to be in place, which is particularly important since a quarter of acute trusts do not yet have a designated stroke unit.

Often there is resistance to setting up stroke services in an acute trust, despite the fact that

Table 1.1: Aim and standards set out in standard 5 of the *National Service Framework*	
Aim	To reduce the incidence of stroke in the population and ensure that those who have had a stroke have prompt access to integrated stroke care services
Standards	The NHS will take action to prevent strokes, working in partnership with other agencies where appropriate
	People who are thought to have had a stroke have access to diagnostic services, are treated appropriately by a specialist stroke service and, subsequently, with their carers, participate in a multidisciplinary programme of secondary prevention and rehabilitation

any one acute hospital site can have as many as thirty-five to forty patients in their beds; stroke patients occupy 20% of hospital beds (Wade, 1994). Setting up a stroke unit can be cost-neutral, and result in increased efficiency, shorter lengths of stay (more people returning to their own residence), reduced mortality and reduced morbidity (Langhorne and Duncan, 2001). The number of stroke patients discharged to their own home within fifty-six days is a benchmark against which trusts are assessed.

Studies from Norway (Indredavik *et al*, 1999) suggest significant savings can be made with improved patient care. The number of patients treated to save one life or disability in the case of stroke units is nine, whereas for some drugs it is a lot higher. For instance, the number needed to treat (NNT) for clopidogrel is between seventy-five and 200 (CAPRIE Steering Committee, 1996; Caro and Migliaccio-Walle, 1999) and for warfarin in atrial fibrillation it is between sixteen and thirty (Koudstaal, 2000). The NNT for antihypertensives is greater depending on patient age. Thrombolysis has a NNT of seven but is only applicable to about 1% of admissions, whereas a stroke unit is applicable to almost all patients with stroke (Lindley, 2002). Interestingly, there is more evidence supporting the use of stroke units than there is for coronary care units.

The NSF is mandatory and gives those people championing stroke a stick with which to beat the drum, along with those provided by the Sentinel Audit and the survey by the British Association of Stroke Physicians (Rodgers *et al*, 2003), both showing that provision of stroke services is woefully inadequate, and in some cases absent. The purpose of all these tools is to deliver high-quality care to all people suffering a stroke.

National Service Framework (NSF)

The NSF has an aim to reduce stroke incidence and to improve stroke care (*Table 1.1*). There are also milestones to be met both for hospital care and general practice (*Tables 1.2* and *1.3*). The NSF details four aspects of stroke care:

1. Prevention.
2. Immediate care.
3. Early and continuing rehabilitation.
4. Long-term care and support.

The aim must be to deliver the same standard of care to all patients irrespective of age and location (postcode). The difference between the standard of care we deliver and that which we would wish to deliver is great — we need to cross that divide.

This article focuses on the management of stroke care around acute phase and rehabilitation. Stroke management is an interagency interdisciplinary problem, not just medical nor just hospital-based.

Table 1.2: Actions set out for the implementation of standard 5

Every health system should, in partnership with other agencies where appropriate:	Review current arrangements, in primary care and elsewhere, to identify those at greatest risk of stroke and to intervene actively to reduce these risks; and agree local priorities to improve rates of identification and effective intervention in stroke
	Review current arrangements, in primary care and elsewhere, for TIA and to agree and implement a local protocol for the rapid referral of patients with TIA who may be at risk of stroke
	Review current hospital services for stroke using the clinical audit methodology developed by the Royal College of Physicians
	On the basis of this, agree local priorities for action to establish an integrated stroke service, which is regularly audited with a continuing cycle of improvement

TIA = transient ischaemic attack

Table 1.3: Milestones for the implementation of stroke care

April 2002	Every general hospital that cares for people with stroke will have plans to introduce a specialist stroke service from 2004	
April 2003	Every hospital that cares for older people with stroke will have established clinical audit systems to ensure delivery of Royal College of Physicians clinical guidelines for stroke	
April 2004	PCTs will have ensured that:	Every general practice, using protocols agreed with local specialist services, can identify and treat patients identified as being at risk of a stroke because of high blood pressure, atrial fibrillation or other risk factors
		Every general practice is using a protocol agreed with local specialist services for the rapid referral and management of those with TIA
		Every general practice can identify people who have had a stroke and is treating them according to protocols agreed with local specialist services
	100% of all general hospitals to have a specialised stroke service in operation	

PCT = primary care trust; TIA = transient ischaemic attack

Immediate care

Acute stroke and transient ischaemic attack (TIA) are medical emergencies. The first challenge is to make the diagnosis and then actively manage to prevent recurrence or deterioration (*Figure*

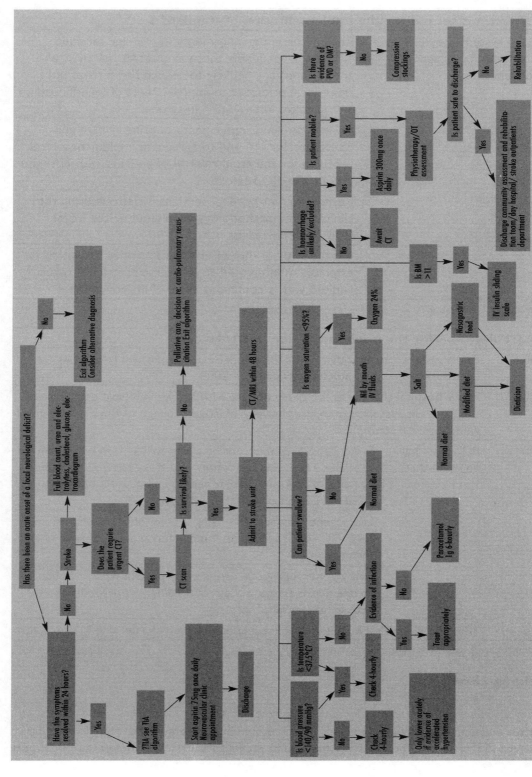

Figure 1.1: Acute care flow chart: East Kent Hospitals algorithm of acute stroke care. BM = finger prick glucose assessment; CT = computed tomography; DM = diabetes mellitus; IV = intravenous; MRI = magnetic resonance imaging; OT = occupational therapy; PVD = peripheral vascular disease; TIA = transient ischaemic attack

1.1). Acute ischaemic stroke should be treated along the same lines as acute ischaemic myocardial damage. The term 'stroke' is slowly being changed to the phrase 'brain attack' suggested by the European Stroke Initiative (Kaste *et al*, 2000).

Changes with neuronal cell permeability can be seen in minutes to hours of stroke onset. A diffusion weighted magnetic resonance imaging scan can show subtle changes very acutely (within minutes), and often there are very subtle changes on the computed tomography scan (loss of definition of the basal ganglia, sulci effacement). Management in the acute phase is about protecting the brain and preventing further neurological damage, and in the case of TIA preventing progression to a completed stroke.

In the acute phase of stroke, the area surrounding the infarct (penumbra) and any haemorrhage (and possibly also in the case of haemorrhage) is potentially salvageable. The penumbra needs protection from further damage. Blood flow below 20 ml/min is unable to maintain neurological function, and at this level the brain autoregulatory system will not work. Protection of the penumbra can be achieved either by restoring blood flow, reducing oedema or reducing toxic free radicals. Neuronal cells die following an infarct. On dying, toxic chemicals are released, including glutamate and aspartamine. Neuroprotective agents bind to the respective receptors to reduce the effect.

Neuronal protection has long been an aim of treatment in the acute phase. There are several approaches, one of which is to stabilise membranes. Many agents have been tried, including antibiotics, steroids, antihypertesives, vitamin E, cannabis derivatives, antiepileptic agents, magnesium, chlormethiazole, naloxone, monoclonal antibodies and hyperbaric oxygen. The IMAGES (Intravenous Magnesium Efficiency in Stroke) study, investigating magnesium, has just finished recruiting and results should be published next year. Many of the neuroprotective agents have failed to show any benefit in man. Whether this is a result of stroke heterogeneity or bad trial design is debated. The other approach is to recanalise the artery that is occluded. Many studies have investigated the role of thrombolytics, aspirin or heparins/heparinoids.

Aspirin

Aspirin (Chinese Acute Stroke Trial, 1997; International Stroke Trial, 1997) has a marginal but positive effect on the acute management of stroke, such that most guidelines suggest giving aspirin at a dose of 300 mg for two weeks, starting within the first forty-eight hours. After this time, the dose can be reduced to between 50 and 300 mg (Intercollegiate Working Party for Stroke, 2000).

Heparin/heparinoids

Many studies have been undertaken using low molecular weight heparins and sodium heparin. Most studies show a reduction in deep vein thrombosis and pulmonary embolus, but this is offset by the increase in symptomatic intracranial haemorrhage. Presently guidelines suggest avoiding heparin in the acute phase of stroke, although there are unanswered questions regarding the use of low-dose subcutaneous sodium heparin.

Thrombolysis

Several agents have undergone clinical trials (recombinant tissue plasminogen activator [rtPA], streptokinase, ancrod, urokinase). Positive results from small studies have been shown with ancrod and vampire-bat saliva, strongly positive results with rtPA, and negative results with streptokinase. Meta-analyses are positive for the use of rtPA, but these rely heavily on one study from the USA. Two large European studies have left the water muddied. These studies (3rd European Cooperative Acute Stroke Study and International Stroke Trial 3; www.dcn. ed.ac.uk/ist3) are investigating the time window for thrombolysis; this is currently less than three hours, and the criteria are strict.

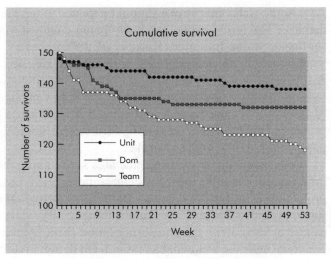

Figure 1.2: Survival following stroke management in different settings. Dom = domicillary

Within the UK, the consensus is that unless a centre is set up to administer, then it should only be used in the context of a trial (Wardlaw, 1998). The British Association of Stroke Physicians are planning to run training programmes for those involved in stroke management who are considering the use of thrombolysis.

Physiological management of acute stroke

Recently, much attention has been paid to 'high tech' management of stroke. An exciting treatment that offers fantastic immediate results often does not come to fruition, or only benefits a small number of patients. It is often blindly accepted that the neurological condition will deteriorate in the first forty-eight hours, and may improve or may not, but this need not be so. Up to 40% of those with an acute stroke undergo 'stroke in progression' and this can often be predicted (Indredavik *et al*, 1999).

Factors that predict or result in progressive neurological damage include increasing age, dehydration, pyrexia, hyperglycaemia, arrhythmia, hypoxia and aspiration. Facilitators of good acute care now accepts that acute management of stroke is proactive, not reactive. Intravenous fluids should be prescribed for the first forty-eight hours, saline not dextrose. Oxygen should be provided if saturations fall below 95%, paracetamol if temperature rises above 37°C, and antibiotics if it rises above 37.5°C. Intravenous insulin should be given if the blood sugar level is >11 mmol/litre (Scott *et al*, 1999).

A raised temperature and a raised blood sugar level are thought to contribute to the ongoing intracranial damage. The evidence for lowering the blood glucose level below 5 mmol/litre is not yet present, although the GIST (Glucose Insulin Stroke Trial) study is being undertaken and coordinated in Sunderland, UK (Scott *et al*, 1999) to investigate this. Certainly, there is evidence of the use of intravenouse insulin to lower glucose from cardiac studies (Malmberg *et al*, 1995).

More radical approaches for the management of acute stroke have examined high-risk patients, especially those with malignant stroke. In these cases, craniotomy may benefit. There is a randomised control study ongoing. There has also been renewed interest in cooling the brain, first reports appearing in the early part of the twentieth century.

Hypertension in the acute phase is more difficult to manage. Current consensus is to observe, and if it remains elevated after the first ten to fourteen days, then to treat. There are no guidelines in this area, but the PROGRESS (Perindopril Protection against Recurrent Stroke) Collaboration Group (2001) and HOPE (Heart Outcomes Prevention Evaluation) (Bosch *et al*, 2002) studies would suggest that an angiotensin-converting enzyme inhibitor would be the agent of first choice, or the second agent to a thiazide. More information is becoming available that supports blockade of the renin–angiotensin system in the wake of recent trials with losartan and canadesartan.

Place of management

Acute phase

Should stroke patients be admitted in the acute phase? Certainly, all patients need to be assessed, probably by an expert and within a short space of time. The Helsingborg declaration (Aboderin and Venables, 1996) suggests that all patients should be assessed by hospital specialists within six hours.

Where should the patient be managed in the acute phase? All the evidence suggests that the best place to be during the acute phase of stroke is an acute stroke unit, which will deliver high-quality care and help reduce death and disability. Ideally, these beds should either be co-located with the rehabilitation unit or be part of the rehabilitation phase. Indredavick's unit is a combined/comprehensive unit with about twenty beds. The maximum length of stay is three weeks, with a median of around eleven days. Most stroke patients have a supported discharge home, others go to a slower rehabilitation facility or stroke unit. The comprehensive stroke unit has a NNT of nine for death and disability, and the positive effect will last for many years (Indredavik *et al*, 1999; Jorgensen *et al*, 2000; Langhorne and Duncan, 2001). Given the lack of acute stroke units in the UK, hospitals need a simple model of care for the acute phase of stroke (*Figure 1.1*) that can be delivered effectively to all stroke patients.

Can the community deliver acute care? People would like to think so, but the evidence says not. Kalra *et al* (2000) conducted a study in the London borough of Bromley, comparing acute in patient management with community management. The stroke unit reduced death and disability compared with the other settings (*Figure 1.2*).

Rehabilitation

Post acute rehabilitation — ie. the first few weeks — is probably best managed in the acute setting (*Table 1.4*). However, after the first ten to twenty-one days, it is appropriate for the right patients to be discharged home with rehabilitation support. Once a patient has been assessed and fully investigated, their rehabilitation can occur at home. The evidence for this is very convincing. People would appear to do at least as well as those that stay in, and maybe better. Many parts of the world are attempting to provide early supported discharge. In the UK, there are models in Devon and Northumberland (www. doh.gov.uk/nsf/olderpeople/index.htm) along these lines, not only using supported discharge but hospitals closer to home for prolonged and slower rehabilitation.

Table 1.4: Early and continuing rehabilitation

Interdiscliplinary working with a multidisciplinary team	Speech therapy	
	Nutritional advice	
	Physiotherapy	
	Occupational therapy	
	Clinical psychology/psychiatry	
	Family support worker	
	Incontinence treatment	
	Equipment/disability aid issues	
Role	Discharge planning	Patient and carer involvement
		Individual care plan
	Objectives	
	Named responsibilities	
	Proposed outcomes	
	Role of stroke care coordinator	
Secondary prevention	Treatment should be initiated in hospital	
	Systems should be in place to ensure treatment is continued in primary care	
	Information given to patients, carers and GPs on treatments	

Despite the evidence, there is a lot of resistance from the public and, in some cases, doctors. Evidence from several trials supports admission for the acute phase then supported discharge, resulting in a short length of stay (Rudd *et al*, 1997; Early Supported Discharge Trialists, 2000).

For those who need rehabilitation after discharge, there has been a focus on rehabilitation at home. This may not suit all. A study in Nottingham, UK, suggested that the frail preferred the day hospital, the young preferred outpatient therapy and those in between preferred to rehabilitate in their own settings (Gladman *et al*, 1993).

When does stroke recovery end? This is a difficult question: it would appear to be many months, if not years, after the initial stroke, but all people are different. Different amounts of improved function will occur at different rates in fairly similar patients. In a nutshell, rehabilitation needs to begin early and continue. For how long is unknown, but certainly it is longer than used to be thought.

Secondary prevention

Management of risk factors is also part of acute or immediate stroke care. Recurrent strokes need to be prevented. Consequently, advice needs to be given regarding a number of areas, including diet (fruit and vegetables, salt and fat intake), cholesterol levels, alcohol intake, exercise, smoking, diabetes, management of hypertension and anticoagulation.

Long-term care

The NSF requires that there should be long-term and ongoing support (*Table 1.5*). The Stroke Association suggests that all patients should be reviewed by their GP within days of discharge. This often does not happen. Long-term follow up is needed to detect changes in patients' clinical, social and psychological condition and their compliance with secondary prevention measures.

Following discharge, many psychological

Table 5.1: Areas for consideration in long-term follow-up

Review following discharge	Short term – 2 months
	Long term – 6 months and annual review
Indications	Action to prevent stroke – secondary prevention
	Reduce death and disability Improved care
	Early, continuing, coordinated rehabilitation
	Long-term support for patients and carers
	Review management plan
Areas to review	Mobility
	Activities of daily living (ADL), personal and extended
	Handicap
	Work
	Driving
	Communication
	Cognitive problems
	Anxiety/depression/memory
	Continence
Further referral	Access to services
	Social services report
	Primary care / secondary care
	Access to specialists
	Stroke coordinators
	Discharge coordinator/clinical nurse specialist
	Family support worker
	Discharge liaison / clinical nurse specialist
	Family support workers
	Maintenance centres
	Stroke clubs

problems may hit (agoraphobia, anxiety, fear, depression) (Robinson, 1998). All patients should be followed up . In many cases, those discharged home are given a follow-up appointment in a clinic, but those in a nursing home often do not get that support. The NSF charges us to review all patients at six months and refer them back to any part of the service that they may need. This is still quite short term; much needs to be done to ensure that patients are reviewed by someone who has good stroke knowledge and, depending on their needs, who can refer them back into the local stroke service. This requires a coordinated response from the health service, social services and often the voluntary sector (*Figure 1.3*). Professionals need to know where to refer for further advice, and patients and carers need to know where to seek advice. This is complex, with a great deal of overlap between services.

These points are not mutually exclusive. If patients are offered ongoing support, then it is possible to identify those that need further review. There are many ways of doing this, including stroke coordinators, liaison nurses, family support workers and informal networks. In Walsall, UK, older patients are followed up by the stroke nurses while younger patients have 'maintenance centres'. Central to all this is the need to maintain a stroke register, which ideally would be nationally based. At present, people moving into an area are missed unless the GP has a practice-based register, as that suggested by projects such as that in East Kent (Primary Care Clinical Effectiveness; www.kentandmedway.nhs.uk/professional_pages/clinical_governance/welcome_to_pricce.asp).

Conclusions

With all the developments in the management of stroke, the future is exciting, and stroke care should be shared between professionals. Simple things will save patients' lives. Good organised care is the way forward: this will save time and lives. Stroke units have a better evidence-base than coronary care units.

The model of stroke care will often depend on local situations. Whichever model is chosen, delivery of acute care with co-located rehabilitation is vital. These units may be next door to each other, in the same department, or in the same clinical area. Both components of hospital care are required if high-quality care is to be delivered. Highly intensive pharmacological therapies could not be administered without acute units.

So often the care of a patient on the ward is variable, depending on the team they are admitted on, which is a disservice. Patients deserve a service where political and historical differences between service providers are laid to rest and where there is joined-up interdisciplinary working that is the best we can deliver, with a determination to make and keep the following promises:

- We will reduce deaths from stroke.
- We will provide a service that will help you reduce your risk of stroke.
- You and your family will be included and supported to make informed decisions about your care and how to prevent stroke.
- You will be offered diagnosis, assessment and treatment by staff who have specialist up-to-date knowledge of stroke.
- We will prevent and treat stroke and TIA using the best and most suitable methods.

References

Aboderin I, Venables G (1996) The Pan European Consensus Meeting on Stroke Management. Stroke Management in Europe. *J Int Med* **240:** 173–80

Bath PM, Willmot MR, Weaver CW, Leanardi-Bee J (2002) Efficacy of nitric oxide in stroke (ENOS) trial: a prospective randomised controlled trial in acute stroke. *Cerebrovasc Dis* **13**(Suppl 3): 8

Bosch J, Yusuf S, Pogue J, *et al* (2002) Use of ramipril in preventing stroke: double-blind randomised control trial. *Br Med J* **324**: 699–704

CAPRIE Steering Committee (1996) A randomised, blinded, trial of clopidogrel versus aspirin in patients at risk of ischaemic events (CAPRIE). *Lancet* **348:** 1329–39

Caro JJ, Migliaccio-Walle K (1999) Generalizable results of clinical trials to actual practice: the example of clopidogrel therapy for the prevention of vascular events. CAPRA (CAPRIE Actual Practice Rate Analysis) Study Group. Clopidogrel vs aspirin in the risk of ischaemic events. *Am J Med* **107:** 568–72

CAST (Chinese Acute Stroke Trial) Collaborative Group (1997) Randomised placebo controlled trial of early aspirin use in 20,000 patients with acute ischaemic stroke. *Lancet* **349:** 1641–9

DoH (2001) *The National Service Framework for Older People.* DoH, London http://www.doh.gov.uk/nsf/olderpeople/index.htm

Early Supported Discharge Trialists (2000) Services for reducing duration of hospital care for acute stroke patients (Cochrane Review). In: The Cochrane Library, Issue 1. Update Software, Oxford

Gladman JRF, Lincoln NB, Barer DH (1993) A randomised controlled trial of domicilary and hospital-based rehabilitation for stroke patients after discharge from hospital. *J Neurol Neurosurg Psychiat* **56:** 960–6

Indredavik B, Bakker F, Slordahl SA, Rokesth R, Haheim LL (1999) Treatment in a combined acute and rehabilitation stroke unit: which aspects are most important. *Stroke* **30:** 793–9

Intercollegiate Working Party for Stroke (2000) *National Clinical Guidelines for Stroke.* Royal College of Physicians, London

Intercollegiate Working Party for Stroke (2001) *Concise Report on the National Sentinel Audit of Stroke 2001–2.* Royal College of Physicians, London

International Stroke Trial Collaborative (1997) The International Stroke Trial (IST): a randomised trial of aspirin, subcutaneous heparin, both or neither among 19,345 patients with acute ischaemic stroke. *Lancet* **349:** 1569–82

Jorgensen HS, Kammersgaard LP, Houth J, *et al* (2000) Who benefits from treatment and rehabilitation in a stroke unit? A community based study. *Stroke* **31:** 434–9

Kalra L, Evans A, Perez I, Kings M, Donaldson N, Swift CG (2000) Alternative strategies to stroke care: a prospective randomised controlled trial. *Lancet* **356:** 894–9

Kaste M, Skyhoj-Olsen T, Orgogozo J-M, Bogousslavsky J, Hacke W for the EUSI Executive Committee (2000) Organization of stroke services. *Cerebrovasc Dis* **10**(S3): 1–4

Koudstaal P (2000) Anticoagulants for preventing stroke in patients with non-rheumatic atrial fibrillation with a history of stroke or transient ischaemic attacks. The Cochrane Library. Update Software, Oxford

Langhorne P, Duncan P (2001) Does the organization of post acute stroke care really matter? *Stroke* **32:** 268

Lindley RI (2002) Thrombolysis for acute stroke in the United Kingdom. *Age Ageing* **31**(S3): 28–30

Malmberg K, Ryden L, Efeendic S, *et al* (1995) Randomised trial of insulin glucose infusion followed by subcutaneous insulin treatment in diabetic patients with acute myocardial infarction (DIGAMI study): effects on mortality at one year. *J Am Coll Cardiol* **26:** 57–65

PROGRESS Collaboration Group (2001) Randomised trial of a perindopril-based blood pressure lowering regimen among 6105 individuals with previous stroke or transient ischaemic attack. *Lancet* **358:** 1033–41

Robinson RG (1998) *The Clinical Neuropsychiatry of Stroke.* Cambridge University Press, Cambridge

Rudd AG, Wolfe CDA, Tilling K, Beech R (1997) Randomised controlled trial to evaluate early discharge scheme for patients with stroke. *BMJ* **315:** 1039–4

Rudd AG, Irwin P, Rutledge Z (1999) The National Sentinel Audit for stroke: a tool for raising standards of care. *J R Coll Physicians Lond* **333:** 460–4

Scott JF, Robinson G, O'Connell JE, Alberti KGMM, Gray CS (1999) Glucose potassium insulin (GKI) infusion in the treatment of acute stroke patients with mild to moderate hyperglycemia (The GIST trial). *Stroke* **30:** 793–9

Wade DT (1994) Stroke (acute cerebrovascular disease). In: Stevens A, Rafferty J (eds) *Health Care Needs Assessment.* Radcliffe Medical Press, Oxford

Wardlaw JM (1998) *RCPE-Consensus Conference on Medical Management of Stroke.* 26–27 May 1998. Background Paper. Royal College of Physicians, Edinburgh

CHAPTER 2

Stroke: implications for practice of the national clinical guidelines

Penny Irwin, Anthony Rudd

The *National Clinical Guidelines for Stroke, 2nd Edition* (Royal College of Physicians, 2004) covers the entirety of stroke management from the time the patient has a transient ischaemic attack (TIA) or stroke right through to living with the longer-term effects. The guidelines' recommendations are based on research evidence and the consensus of the intercollegi~ate stroke working party responsible for their development. They are also influenced by the views of patients and carers, which were obtained in focus groups (Kelson *et al*, 1998) conducted to inform the first edition of the guidelines (Royal College of Physicians, 2000) and more recent qualitative research (McKevitt and Wolfe, 2004). The method used to grade the recommendations and strength of the evidence supporting them is displayed in *Table 2.1*.

Table 2.1: Level of evidence and grade of recommendation

Level of evidence	Type of evidence	Grade of recommendation
Ia	Meta-analysis of randomised controlled trials (RCTs)	A
Ib	At least one RCT	A
IIa	At least one well-designed, controlled study but without randomisation	B
IIb	At least one well-designed, quasi-experimental study	B
III	At least one well-designed, non-experimental descriptive study (eg. comparative studies, correlation studies, case studies)	B
IV	Expert committee reports, opinions and/or experience of respected authorities.	C
Working party consensus	Recommended good practice based on the clinical experience of the Guideline Group	D

The model for care

Stroke is one of the most devastating disorders. It varies from a minor momentary transient ischaemic attack (TIA), which resolves within 24 hours, to a major stroke, which leaves the person with profound physical disabilities and cognitive deficits that change them forever. It kills a third of those it strikes, and is the country's highest cause of major disability. The guidelines therefore cover an immense diversity of problems. The World Health Organisation's (WHO) *International Classification of Functioning, Disability and Health* (WHO, 2001) provides a useful framework for the management of conditions with such long-term effects:

• pathology — disease at the organ/system level eg. the part of the brain affected by the stroke
• impairment — the signs and symptoms on the body eg. hemiplegia, dysphasia
• activity — function or observed behaviour of the person in their environment eg. difficulty walking as a result of the hemilpegia
• participation/handicap — the effect of illness on the social roles of the person (eg. work, caring for children, etc).

The model also takes into account the personal experiences, and the social and physical environment of the person. Within this framework, the guidelines focus on the patient's problems, and rehabilitation seeks to maximise the person's sense of well-being, while minimising distress. The content is organised into four main sections:

• service provision
• acute management
• rehabilitation
• transfer to community.

Service provision

Because the evidence is so strong that patients with stroke have better outcomes if they are managed in a stroke unit (Stroke Unit Triallists' Collaboration, 2002), the first section of the guidelines concentrates on all aspects of service provision. In the four years since the first edition, evidence has emerged showing a much higher risk of stroke after TIA than previously thought. Similarly, immediately after stroke the need to control physiological parameters such as temperature, blood sugar and oxygen levels to prevent worse outcomes has become more widely accepted. The guidelines recommend that hospitals offer enhanced specialist services in the form of:

▪ Specialist neurovascular clinics that can investigate patients within a week of TIA.
▪ Acute stroke units that provide continuous monitoring in the early days after stroke, so adverse signs and symptoms can be more effectively controlled.

With the advent of the licensing of the drug alteplase for thrombolysis after ischaemic stroke, services offering this intervention have to be registered with the international audit — Safe Implementation of Thrombolysis in Stroke Monitoring Study (SITS-MOST). To maximise the number of patients eligible for thrombolysis, centres should have special systems in place. These include arrangements with the ambulance service for stroke to be treated as an emergency, so that patients are transferred to the specialist centre for treatment within three hours of their stroke.

Even in areas where thrombolysis is not available, with the evidence so strongly showing better outcomes for patients who are treated in a stroke unit after stroke, it is now recommended that all patients suspected of having had a stroke are referred to hospital for investigation and management. The unit should include all the disciplines and equipment necessary to provide a comprehensive service for acute management and rehabilitation. The results from each round of the National Sentinel Audit of Stroke (Rudd *et al*, 1999; Rudd *et al*, 2001; Irwin, 2004) show that patients cared for in general wards receive inferior care compared with those who receive stroke unit care, and the mortality rates are lower in those hospitals that treat higher proportions of cases in their stroke units (Rudd *et al*, 2004). Similarly, in the community, patients managed by non-specialist teams have worse outcomes than those managed in hospital stroke units or by specialist community rehabilitation teams (Early Supported Discharge Trialists, 2004; Ronning and Guldvog, 1998; Outpatient Service Trialists, 2004). *The National Clinical Guidelines for Stroke* (Royal College of Physicians, 2004: 13–17) therefore recommend that patients should only be discharged early from hospital if managed by a specialist team.

■ Specialist stroke services should be available in the community, as part of an integrated system of care to facilitate early supported discharge (A).
■ Specialist day hospital rehabilitation or specialist domiciliary rehabilitation can be offered to outpatients with equal effect (A).

National Clinical Guidelines for Stroke, 2nd Edition (2004: 13–17)

Palliative care

Effective management of the dying patient is as important as active management of those less severely affected. Guidelines are therefore included on palliative care. There was little research evidence specific to stroke to support these, but the NICE (2004) guidelines on palliative cancer and the BMA publication *Witholding and Withdrawing Life-Prolonging Medical Treatment* (BMA, 2002) offered helpful guidance for this difficult area.

a. All staff providing palliative care for patients after stroke should be trained in the principles and practice of palliative care (D).
b. All stroke patients should have access to specialist palliative care expertise when needed (D).
c. End of life decisions to withhold or withdraw life-prolonging treatments (including artificial nutrition and hydration) should be in the best interests of the patient (D).

National Clinical Guidelines for Stroke, 2nd Edition (2004: 25)

Acute care

Acute TIA

It is now known that up to 20% of those suffering a TIA will have a stroke within a month, with a high likelihood of it occurring within seven days. The guidelines therefore recommend that patients should be referred to a specialist neurovascular clinic within seven days, in the meantime being started on an antiplatelet agent immediately, with other risk factors (eg. severe hypertension) urgently reviewed and treatment begun. If patients are diagnosed as having more than 70% carotid stenosis, it is recommended that carotid endarterectomy should be performed in a specialist centre, preferably within two weeks of TIA for maximum benefit, and certainly within twelve weeks for any benefit (Williams *et al*, 2004).

Investigation and management of acute stroke

Evidence on the management of acute stroke is rapidly evolving, showing it should be managed much more actively than had previously been thought, and how vital it is to ensure that the proper diagnosis is made through early imaging, particularly if haemorrhage is suspected, or thrombolysis is an option. If subarachnoid haemorrhage is diagnosed, the patient should be immediately transferred to a neurosurgical centre.

All patients should be assessed for risks of complications that could hinder their recovery (eg. for dysphagia, risk of developing pressure sores, deep vein thromboses) and managed accordingly. Continuous physiological monitoring is recommended to allow management of adverse signs in the early days after stroke (eg. temperature, blood sugar and oxygen levels, hydration). The guidelines on the management of bladder and bowel problems discourage the early use of indwelling catheters, promoting active management in preference.

There has been a lot of research into drugs that could salvage ischaemic brain (eg. neuroprotectors and drugs to reduce cerebral oedema) and protect the brain from further damage after stroke. Sadly, there is no evidence to support the use of any drugs for routine use in this area. The main emphasis is, therefore, on secondary prevention being started as soon as possible. Patients with ischaemic stroke should be prescribed antithrombotic treatment (eg. aspirin 300mg) to be commenced within the first forty-eight hours.

Secondary prevention

Following a stroke, patients are at significant increased risk of a further stroke (30–43% within five years). They are also at risk of other vascular events such as myocardial infarction and peripheral vascular disease. The evidence that secondary prevention is effective is overwhelming. Effective secondary prevention includes providing sensible lifestyle advice and support to those with obesity, hyperlipidaemia, nicotine and alcohol addiction, and requires all those in the front line of health care to encourage concordance with anti-hypertensive, anti-thrombotic or lipid-lowering medication.

Tight control of blood pressure within the limits set by the British Hypertension Society (Williams *et al*, 2004) is the single most important component of secondary prevention. There is little evidence that any particular anti-hypertensive drug is better than any other. The key point is to find one that is effective and acceptable to the patient. Ischaemic stroke should be treated with either anti-platelet drugs or anti-coagulants. Anti-platelet therapy should either be aspirin alone (75mg daily from two weeks after stroke) or another anti-platelet agent. Where patients are aspirin intolerant, clopidogrel or dipyridamole are recommended. Whether to use warfarin for patients with atrial fibrillation or recent myocardial infarction needs to be decided for each individual patient. The evidence from the trials is unequivocal: it is beneficial. Unfortunately, the trials did not include many of the older, frailer patients, where the risks of anticoagulation (falls or difficulty with concordance) outweigh their benefit. In these cases, anti-platelet drugs should be substituted.

The frequent need for multiple medications has implications for concordance when patients return home. It is therefore important that they are given written information with education about their medication, and supplied with compliance aids appropriate to their needs and preferences (Royal College of Physicians, 2004: 44).

Rehabilitation

Teamworking

To enable all disciplines to work together with the patient in a consistent way during rehabilitation, the NCG guidelines recommend that they meet regularly (at least once a week) to review patients' progress. They should also have an agreed approach to therapy and assessment measures, with goals set at the team level.

- All members of the healthcare team should work together with the patient, carer and family, using a shared philosophy and common goals (B).
- Any of the current therapeutic approaches to movement re-education should be used to improve function (A).
- Goals should be set at the team level, as well as at the level of an individual clinician (D).

National Clinical Guidelines for Stroke, 2nd Edition (2004: 23)

Evidence is growing regarding the value of high-intensity therapy, so in the second edition of the *National Clinical Guidelines for Stroke*, the importance of patients having the opportunity to practice the skills and activities learned in therapy sessions is emphasised.

- The team should promote the practice of skills gained in therapy into the patient's daily routine in a consistent manner (A).

National Clinical Guidelines for Stroke, 2nd Edition (2004: 24)

Mood disorders

Mood disorders after stroke, including emotionalism (which usually presents as persistent tearfulness but may include inappropriate laughter), anxiety and depression are common. It is recognised that depression may be a transitory phase that resolves without treatment, but these patients require careful observation, so that those who do not get better can be prescribed the appropriate treatment, and referred for specialist advice to a psychiatrist or clinical psychologist where necessary.

Cognitive deficits

Cognitive impairments are amongst the hardest to recognise after stroke. Although there is increasing research in areas such as spatial awareness, attention, memory, praxis and executive function (Williams *et al*, 2004; Rothwell *et al*, 2004; Bowen *et al*, 2004; Lincoln *et al*, 2004; Majid *et al*, 2004), there is still a need for much more research on the management of the problems they bring. In the service organisation section, the guidelines therefore recommend a clinical psychologist is a member of the stroke team. The section specific to this problem then shows that all members need to be alert to the possibilities of cognitive impairments and knowledgeable in methods of screening so they can refer those requiring more in-depth assessment to the psychologist.

- All patients should be screened for the presence of cognitive impairments as soon as is practicable. The nature of the impairment should be determined, and its impact on activity and participation should be explained to patients, carers and staff (D).
- Those with difficulty on screening, and anyone not progressing as expected in rehabilitation, should have a detailed assessment (D).

National Clinical Guidelines for Stroke, 2nd Edition (2004: 56)

Communication disorders

Aphasia requires speech and language therapy from an expert speech and language therapist. The value of the family's support with the help from other members of the team is also recognised as essential to the patient's efforts to communicate. Sometimes group sessions may also be helpful for those with longer-term aphasia.

- If the patient has aphasia, the staff and relatives should be informed and trained by the speech and language therapist about communication techniques appropriate to the communication disability (A).
- For patients with long-term aphasia, a period of speech and language therapy intervention, including group communication treatment, should be considered (A).

National Clinical Guidelines for Stroke, 2nd Edition (2004: 60)

Mobility

Early mobilisation after stroke is one of the key elements of stroke unit care. Physiotherapy research is beginning to show the advantages of particular techniques to overcome the movement problems that occur with stroke. This requires a physiotherapist with particular expertise in neuro-rehabilitation to be a member of the team so that appropriate interventions are started as soon as possible.

- A physiotherapist with expertise in neuro-disability should coordinate therapy to improve movement performance of patients with stroke (C).
- Intensive therapy for the upper limb should be considered to improve arm function in patients with mild impairment (A).
- Gait-re-education techniques to improve walking ability that are based on recognised therapy approaches should be offered to improve walking ability (B).
- Treadmill training (with partial body-weight support) should not be used on a routine basis (A).
- Resisted exercise should be considered to improve muscle strength in targeted muscles (A).
- Patients should participate in cardiovascular training (aerobic activity) (A).

National Clinical Guidelines for Stroke, 2nd Edition (2004: 62–8)

Some of the newer techniques being used in research trials are gaining credible amounts of evidence, such as treadmill training with body-weight support (Moseley *et al*, 2004) or constraint induced movement therapy for the upper limb (Van der Lee *et al*, 1999; Dromerick *et al*, 2000). However, the evidence seems to show they are suitable only for distinct groups of patients. Those providing therapies at service level also have to consider factors such as the costs of equipment against the benefit, as well as the preferences of patients.

- For patients who can walk independently, treadmill training with partial body-weight support (>40%) between thirty days to three months post-stroke should be considered as an adjunct to conventional therapy (B).
- Constraint-induced therapy to increase the use of the affected arm should be considered in patients with at least ten degrees of active wrist and finger extension, who are more than a year post-stroke and who can walk independently without an aid (B).

National Clinical Guidelines for Stroke, 2nd Edition (2004: 64, 68)

The recommendations for ankle foot orthoses to improve walking ability include that they be individually fitted. Serial casting is recommended to reverse contractures and reduce spasticity.

Sensory impairment and pain

Central post-stroke pain is a distressing complication that may arise after stroke, and which may not be recognised by staff unused to the condition. The recommendations are:

- Neuropathic pain may respond to tricyclic antidepressants (eg. amitriptyline) or anticonvulsants (eg. gabapentin) (A).
- Patients with intractable pain should be referred to a specialist pain service as soon as possible (D).

National Clinical Guidelines for Stroke, 2nd Edition (2004: 68–70)

Functional activity

The coordination of therapy to help the patient perform simple everyday tasks so that they can manage at home is the role of the specialist occupational therapist. This may require equipment or adaptations to the patient's home so they can function more effectively.

- All patients with difficulties in activities of daily living (ADL) should be assessed by an occupational therapist with specialist knowledge in neurological rehabilitation (A).
- Patients should be supplied as soon as possible with all aids, adaptations and equipment they need (A).
- Every patient who is at home or leaving hospital should be assessed fully to determine whether equipment or adaptations can increase safety or independence (A).
- The suitability and use of equipment should be reviewed over time as needs will change (B).
- All patients should be given a contact number for future advice or help with equipment provided (D).

National Clinical Guidelines for Stroke, 2nd Edition (2004: 72–5)

The occupational therapist will also have a key role in helping the team work with the patient to overcome problems associated with cognitive impairments, particularly in centres where a clinical psychologist is not included in the team. Their advice may also prove helpful in working with patients to develop strategies so they remember the medications they need to take for secondary prevention.

Transfer to community

Because patient and carer focus groups and research show how isolated and abandoned people feel once they leave hospital after stroke (Royal College of Physicians, 1998, 2000), the guidelines cover the management of problems after transfer to the community, taking into account patients' possible needs for further rehabilitation, secondary prevention and social support.

a. Early hospital discharge to generic (non-specialist) community services should not be undertaken (A).
b. Carers should receive all necessary equipment and training in moving and handling, in order to position and transfer the patient safely in the home environment (B).
c. Patients should continue to have access to specialist stroke care and rehabilitation after leaving hospital (A).

National Clinical Guidelines for Stroke, 2nd Edition (2004: 77–8)

Rehabilitation long-term after stroke

It is often a cause of distress to patients after stroke that their therapy is stopped when they feel they still need more. The guidelines highlight the benefit of therapy starting again late after stroke, but recommend proper assessment. They also show the need for patients to regain their independence and for treatments to be withdrawn in a planned way.

▪ Any patient with reduced activity at six months or later after stroke should be assessed for a period of further targeted rehabilitation (A).
▪ Independence should be encouraged. As patients become more active, consideration should be given to withdrawal of physical and psychological support, enteral tubes, cessation of therapy and withdrawal of personal care support (D).

National Clinical Guidelines for Stroke, 2nd Edition (2004: 79)

Secondary prevention in primary care

Secondary prevention of stroke begins in the acute phase straight after stroke. It then continues lifelong. The risk factors will require close monitoring and medications prescribed accordingly (the detailed recommendations for secondary prevention have been brought together in a *Concise Guide for Primary Care*). It is part of the GP contract that they should know which patients on their lists have had a stroke and routinely monitor their condition.

Social support

Research shows the extent and nature of the stress of caring for a disabled person and the factors influencing it (Nolan *et al*, 1995, 1996; Pound *et al*, 1999). Carers and families may need long-term practical, emotional, social and financial support to cope with the many residual problems after stroke.

The recommendations stress the importance of giving good-quality information, both written and verbal and follow the evidence which suggests the importance of educational strategies in combination with information giving. As with the first edition of the guidelines, a patient and carer information booklet (Royal College of Physicians, 2004b) based on the guidelines is available either from the Royal College of Physicians or through the Stroke Association Helpline. This also contains information about patients' and carers' support organisations who provide information on the different aspects of life after stroke and the services available (see websites at the end of the chapter).

- Information provision should take into account the needs of each individual (D).
- Information should be freely available to patients and their families in a variety of languages and formats specific to patient impairments (A).
- Patients and carers should be offered education programmes to assist them in adapting to their new role (B).
- Stroke services must be alert to the likely stress on carers, specifically recognising the stress associated with 'hidden' impairments such as cognitive loss, urinary incontinence, and irritability (B).

National Clinical Guidelines for Stroke, 2nd Edition (2004: 19–20)

Childhood stroke

Because of the popular belief that stroke is a disease of old age and does not happen in childhood, children who suffer a stroke are liable to receive poor standards of care by non-specialist staff. Following requests from patients' groups and concerned professionals, it was agreed that the second edition of the adult guidelines would be accompanied by guidelines for the diagnosis, management and rehabilitation of stroke in childhood (Royal College of Physicians, 2004c). The evidence-base for these was not as strong as it is for stroke in adults. However, the guidelines bring together such research as there is, the key Government policy documents on the management of children living with long-term conditions, and consensus statements on appropriate management. It is hoped this will not only help improve standards of care for these children and their families, but also stimulate further research into all aspects of childhood stroke. A parent information booklet (Paediatric Stroke Working Party: Royal College of Physicians, 2004d) accompanies the guidelines and is available from the Stroke Association Helpline.

Conclusion

The National Clinical Guidelines for Stroke were first published in 2000 after years of patchy service provision for one of the country's most common conditions. The results of the National Sentinel Audit of Stroke every two years show services are gradually improving but we still have a long way to go for all patients to receive first class evidence based care. The second edition of the guidelines in 2004 gives further guidance to that goal.

References

Bowen A, Lincoln N, Dewey M (2004) Cognitive rehabilitation for spatial neglect following stroke (Cochrane Review). In: The Cochrane Library, Issue 1, 2004. John Wiley & Sons, Chichester

British Medical Association (2002) *Witholding and Withdrawing Life-Prolonging Medical Treatment: Guidance for Decision Making*. 2nd edn. BMJ Books, London

Donkervoort M, Dekker J, Stehmann-Saris F, Deelman B (2001) Efficacy of strategy training in left hemisphere stroke patients with apraxia: a randomized clinical trial. *Neuropsychol Rehabil* **11**: 549–66

Dromerick A, Edwards D, Hahn M (2000) Does the application of constraint induced movement therapy during acute rehabilitation reduce arm impairment after ischaemic stroke? *Stroke* **31**: 2984–8

Early Supported Discharge Trialists (2004). Services for reducing duration of hospital care for acute stroke patients (Cochrane Review). In: The Cochrane Library, Issue 3, 2004. John Wiley & Sons, Chichester

Intercollegiate Working Party for Stroke (2000) *National Clinical Guidelines for Stroke*. Royal College of Physicians, London

Intercollegiate Stroke Working Party (2004) *National Clinical Guidelines for Stroke*. 2nd edn. Royal College of Physicians, London

Intercollegiate Working Party for Stroke (2004b) *Care after Stroke and Transient Ischaemic Attack: Information for Patients and their Carers*. Royal College of Physicians, London

Irwin P, Hoffman A, Lowe D, Pearson MG, Rudd AG (2004) Improving clinical practice in stroke through audit: results of three rounds of national stroke audit. *J Eval Clin Pract* (in press)

Kelson M, Ford C, Rigge M (1998) *Stroke Rehabilitation: Patient and Carer Views: a Report by the College of Health for the Intercollegiate Working Party for Stroke*. Royal College of Physicians, London

Lincoln N, Majid M, Weyman N (2004) Cognitive rehabilitation for attention deficits following stroke (Cochrane Review). In: The Cochrane Library, Issue 1, 2004. John Wiley & Sons,

Chichester

Majid M, Lincoln N, Weyman N (2004) Cognitive rehabilitation for memory deficits following stroke (Cochrane Review). In: The Cochrane Library, Issue 1, 2004. John Wiley & Sons, Chichester

McKevitt C, Wolfe C (2004) *An Anthropological Investigation of Lay and Professional Meanings of Quality of Life.* Economic and Social Research Council, Swindon

Moseley A, Stark A, Cameron I, Pollock A (2004) Treadmill training and body weight support for walking after stroke (Cochrane Review). In: The Cochrane Library, Issue 1, 2004. John Wiley & Sons, Chichester

National Institute for Clinical Excellence (NICE) (2004) Supportive and palliative care for people with cancer: Part A and Part B. National Institute for Clinical Excellence, London

Nolan M, Keady J, Grant G (1995) Developing a typology of family care: implications for nurses and other service providers. *J Adv Nurs* **21**: 256–65

Nolan M, Walker G, Nolan J, Williams S, Poland F, Curran M, Kent BC (1996) Entry to care: positive choice or fait accompli? Developing a more proactive nursing response to the needs of older people and their carers. *J Adv Nurs* **24**: 265–74

Outpatient Service Trialists (2004) Therapy-based rehabilitation services for stroke patients at home (Cochrane Review). In: The Cochrane Library, Issue 3, 2004. John Wiley & Sons, Chichester

Paediatric Stroke Working Party (2004c) *Stroke in Childhood: Clinical Guidelines for Diagnosis, Management and Rehabilitation.* Royal College of Physicians, London

Paediatric Stroke Working Party (2004d) *Care After Stroke in Childhood: Information for Parents and Families of Children Affected by Stroke.* Royal College of Physicians, London

Pound P, Gompertz, Ebrahim S (1999) Social and practical strategies described by people living at home with stroke. *Health Soc Care Community* **7**(2): 120–6

Ronning O, Guldvog B (1998) Outcome of subacute stroke rehabilitation: a randomized controlled trial. *Stroke* **29**: 779–84

Rothwell P, Eliasziw M, Gutnikov S *et al* and Carotid Endarterectomy Trialists Collaboration (2004) Endarterectomy for symptomatic carotid stenosis in relation to clinical subgroups and timing of surgery. *Lancet* **363**: 915–24

Rudd AG, Hoffman A, Irwin P, Pearson M, Lowe D (2004) Stroke unit care and outcome. Results from the 2001 National Sentinel Audit of Stroke (England, Wales and Northern Ireland). *Stroke* **Nov 29**: Epub ahead of print.

Rudd AG, Irwin P, Rutledge Z, Lowe D, Morris R, Pearson MG (1999) The National Sentinel Audit of Stroke: a tool for raising standards of care. *J R Coll Physicians Lond* **30**: 460–4

Rudd AG, Irwin P, Rutledge Z, Lowe D, Pearson MG (2001) National stroke audit: a tool for change? *Qual Health Care* **10**: 141–51

Stroke Unit Triallists' Collaboration (2004) Organised inpatient (stroke unit) care for stroke (Cochrane Review). In: The Cochrane Library, Issue 3, 2004. John Wiley & Sons, Chichester

Van der Lee J, Wagenaar R, Lankhorst G, Vogelaar T *et al* (1999) Forced use of the upper extremity in chronic stroke patients: results from a single-blind randomised clinical trial. *Stroke* **30**: 2369–75

Williams B, Poulter N, Brown M, Davies M *et al* (2004) Guidelines for management of hypertension: report of the fourth working party of the British Hypertension Society 2004 BHS IV. *J Hum Hypertens* **18**: 139–85

Wilson B, Emslie H, Quirk K, Evans J (2001) Reducing everyday memory and planning problems by means of a paging system: a randomised control crossover study. *J Neurol Neurosurg Psychiatry* **70**: 477–82

World Health Organisation (WHO) (2001) *International Classification of Functioning Disability and Health*. WHO, Geneva

Useful websites and addresses

Royal College of Physicians	www.rcplondon.ac.uk
SITS-MOST	www.acutestroke.org
Stroke Association	www.stroke.org.uk
Chest Heart Stroke Scotland	www.chss.org.uk
Different Strokes	www.differentstrokes.co.uk
NICHSA	www.nichsa.com
Connect	www.ukconnect.org
Speakability	www.speakability.org.uk

CHAPTER 3

Evidence-based guidelines for early stroke management

Majnu Pushpangadan, John Wright, John Young

Stroke disease is the commonest neurological emergency encountered by the junior medical team. We have reviewed the literature to produce a series of substantiated guidelines to assist the admitting doctor in managing early stroke care optimally.

Stroke is a common medical emergency. Almost 25% of men and 20% of women at forty-five years of age can expect to have a stroke if they live to be eighty-five years old (Bonita, 1992). Concepts and management of patients with stroke have changed considerably in recent years and there is evidence that optimal care is inconsistently applied (Lindley *et al*, 1995a, 1995b). Although many reviews of stroke care are available, their format has been largely discursive, concerned with informing rather than providing clinical guidelines aimed at reducing variability in clinical practice.

Clinical guidelines are effective in improving the quality and outcomes of patient care (Grimshaw and Russell, 1993; Effective Health Care, 1994) and reducing variations in practice. Our aim has been to develop evidence-based guidelines for early stroke care, principally to assist decision-making for the admitting junior doctor. These guidelines cover the first twenty-four hours of care, when inconsistent clinical decision-making is common and may not be easily corrected later.

Scope of the guidelines

The guidelines are based on the World Health Organisation's (WHO) definition of stroke:

> *A syndrome of rapidly developing clinical signs of focal (or global) disturbance of cerebral function, with symptoms lasting twenty-four hours or longer or leading to death with no apparent cause other than of vascular origin.*
>
> WHO, MONICA Project Principal Investigators (1988)

They are not therefore comprehensive for transient ischaemic attack (TIA) management. We have also excluded 'young' patients with stroke (arbitrarily defined as <forty-five years), as the underlying causal mechanisms are more varied and conventional vascular risk-factors less prominent (Martin *et al*, 1997). Inevitably, there is some blurring of the selected timeframe and some of the guidelines go beyond the first twenty-four hours (eg. management of atrial fibrillation [AF] or hypertension). This is simply to reflect natural clinical processes and to provide guidelines that are clinically relevant. However, certain important but less immediate stroke issues such as nutritional support for persisting dysphagia, and the whole area of rehabilitation, have not been addressed.

Finally, we have assumed an acute medical ward or a medical admission unit as the setting in which these guidelines will be applied. Although well-coordinated stroke care in stroke rehabilitation units provides superior outcome to stroke care on general medical wards (Stroke Unit Triallists Collaboration, 1997), the benefit of specialised acute stroke units is unclear (Bath *et al*, 1996).

Method

A series of Medline (1966–1998) searches using key words and subject headings was used to identify relevant articles. This was supplemented by searches of the Stroke Module of the Cochrane Library up to June, 1998. The information obtained and the resulting guideline has been classified according to accepted levels of evidence:

- Level A: based on randomised controlled trials (RCT) or meta-analysis of RCTs
- Level B: based on robust experimental or observational studies
- Level C: based on expert opinion.

Wherever possible, we have sought RCT evidence and especially systematic reviews of RCTs for our guidelines, as this method provides the least biased and most precise information.

A guidelines development group was convened to review the evidence. This comprised consultant staff from neurology, care of the elderly, general medicine, radiology and public-health medicine.

Recommendations were based on the strength of the evidence and its applicability to local circumstances. Informal consensus methods were used to agree recommendations.

Review of the guidelines was undertaken by consultant medical staff in the hospital. A three-month period for piloting the guidelines took place. They were subsequently reappraised and modified in the light of feedback from medical staff.

History and examination

A stroke clerking proforma has been developed as a basis for clinical audit (Royal College of Physicians, 1994). Although this approach can improve the completeness of patient assessment

(Davenport *et al*, 1995), it is unclear whether improved management and outcomes are achieved.

History

Despite advances in neuroradiology the diagnosis of stroke remains primarily a clinical one. The WHO definition of stroke emphasises the importance of a history which uncovers a sudden onset neurological deficit. If the patient is unable to give a history (reduced consciousness, dysphasia, dementia), then a witness account should be specifically sought as this improves the precision of the diagnosis (Sandercock *et al*, 1985; Allen, 1993). Indeed, a history and examination has a sensitivity of 95% (only 5% false negative diagnosis) but a more variable specificity of 66–97% (3%–34% false positive diagnosis), with the higher percentage representing more experienced clinicians (Ebrahim, 1990).

It is good practice while taking the history to identify the person behind the stroke by understanding their pre-stroke lifestyle, housing and family structure. Pre-stroke disability can be assessed using the Barthel Index (Mahoney and Barthel, 1965). This background is valuable in informing the appropriateness of potential treatments and promotes a process of support and interest which patients value during the crisis stage of stroke (Pound *et al*, 1995).

Guideline 1 (level B)

A careful history is reliable in the diagnosis of stroke. Patient and/or their family should be informed about the diagnosis of stroke and given the opportunity of asking questions.

Examination

The purpose of examination at presentation is to secure further the diagnosis of stroke, specify the impairments, identify the subtype of ischaemic stroke (Bamford *et al*, 1991; Anderson *et al*, 1994) (*Table 3.1*) and identify co-existing conditions such as chronic respiratory disease, cardiac failure and peripheral vascular disease. Stroke subclassification is important because it gives useful indication of prognosis for early mortality, recurrence and functional outcome (*Table 3.2*). Examination at maximal neurological deficit also identifies associated important features in early management, eg. impaired consciousness, impaired swallow, initial blood pressure (BP), presence of AF, fever and hypoxia. The former two issues are discussed here and the others later in the text.

- ❖ **Consciousness:** Impaired consciousness can be quantified using the Glasgow Coma Score. A reduced coma score is associated with a worse outcome in acute stroke (Oxbury *et al*, 1975). Although sepsis and metabolic factors may contribute to drowsiness, impaired consciousness generally indicates the presence of cerebral oedema with associated raised intracranial pressure (Roper and Shafran, 1984).

❖ **Swallowing:** Unsafe swallowing may affect up to a third of stroke patients on admission. About a half will recover within the first week but about 10% will have persisting impairment at one month (Barer, 1989). An immediate assessment of swallowing in conscious patients is important to determine the risk of aspiration. Testing the gag reflex is unhelpful as it does not discriminate between safe and unsafe swallowing (Horner *et al*, 1988; Davies *et al*, 1995).

Table 3.1: The Oxford classification of cerebral infarction

TACI	Hemi motor and sensory deficit
	Hemianopia
	Cortical dysfunction Dysphasia
	Visuospatial disturbance
PACI	Any two of the above (eg. dysphasia and hemiplegia) or an isolated cortical dysfunction (eg. dysphasia)
LACI	Pure motor hemiplegia
	Pure sensory loss
	Motor and sensory loss
POCI	Vertigo, diplopia, ataxia, isolated hemianopia

Table 3.2: Outcomes according to cerebral infarct clinical symptoms

	30-day mortality	3-month recurrence	6-month dependence
TACI	39%	Low	39%
PACI	4%	Very high	34%
LACI	2%	Low	26%
POCI	7%	High	18%

LACI = lacunar infarction; PACI = partial anterior (=carotid) circulation infarct; POCI = posterior circulation infarction; TACI = total anterior (=carotid) circulation infarct

Videofluoroscopy, widely accepted as the 'gold standard' for swallowing assessment, is impractical for routine use in the acute stroke setting. A simple bedside evaluation is the preferred approach and should be routinely employed using a standardised swallowing assessment (Splaincard *et al*, 1988; Kidd *et al*, 1993; Smithard *et al*, 1996), one example of which is given in *Figure 3.1*. Using a pulse oximeter to detect desaturation during swallowing as a predictive marker for aspiration has been described but needs further study (Zaidi *et al*, 1995; Collins and Bakheit, 1997).

Guideline 2 (level B)

Examination at presentations should describe the neurological impairments and identify the stroke sub-type. Assessment of consciousness and swallowing should always be recorded.

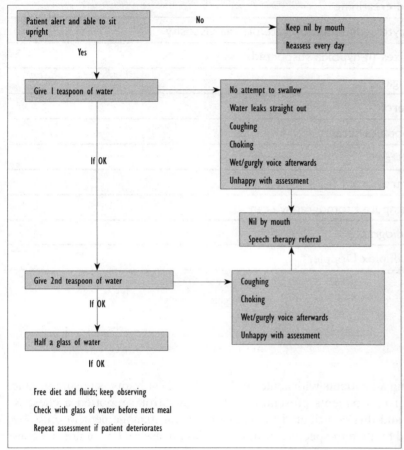

Figure 3.1: Standardised swallowing assessment

Cardiopulmonary resuscitation status

After the history and examination, the most senior doctor available should make a decision on the cardiopulmonary resuscitation (CPR) status of the patient. The pre-stroke disability and lifestyle assessment is important in informing the CPR status. Resuscitation is rarely successful (and therefore generally inappropriate) in patients who have impaired consciousness from a major stroke (Schneider *et al*, 1993).

Guideline 3 (level B):

CPR status should be clearly recorded in the case notes with a date for review.

Investigations

The investigation of acute stroke should be directed towards delineating the type of stroke (infarct or haemorrhage), candidate causes and uncovering risk factors for future vascular events (*Table 3.3*). A full blood count will detect anaemia (exacerbates cerebral hypoxia) and conditions associated with vascular stasis (erythrocytosis or thrombocytosis). Measurement of plasma viscosity or erythrocyte sedimentation rate may direct the physician towards a vasculitis, particularly cranial arteritis. Patients with no vascular risk factors and a history of venous or arterial thrombosis should be investigated for a thrombophilia (clotting screen, protein C & S). Blood glucose and cholesterol are discussed later in the text.

Table 3.3: Investigations in suspected cases of acute stroke

Blood	Full blood count
	Urea and creatinine
	Erythrocyte sedimentation rate/plasma viscosity
	Blood gases (if hypoxia suspected)
	Blood sugar
	Cholesterol
	Thrombophilia screen*
Radiological/ cardiological	Chest X-ray*
	Electrocardiogram
	Head computed tomography scan
	Echocardiography*
	Carotid duplex Doppler*

*Selected patients only (see text)

Chest X-ray

A clinical policy of investigating all patients with acute stroke with a chest X-ray is unsupportable. A study (Sagar *et al*, 1996) of 435 patients presenting with a new stroke reported a chest X-ray abnormality in only 16% and this contributed to changed clinical management in only 4%. Although the study was limited by its retrospective design, and did not assess how a normal chest X-ray appearance might influence management, it seems sensible to request the investigation only in the presence of specific indications such as weight loss or unexplained chest symptoms.

Guideline 4 (level B)

A routine chest X-ray is unnecessary.

Electrocardiogram

Stroke and heart disease share common epidemiological and clinicopathological features. A cardiac cause of death following stroke is not uncommon during the first month (Ebrahim, 1990).

An electrocardiogram (ECG) will reliably identify AF (see later) and can indicate pre-existing ischaemic heart disease (eg. Q waves), both of which have important implications for secondary vascular prevention or for rehabilitation (Roth, 1994).

Guideline 5 (level B)

All conscious stroke patients should have an ECG.

Head computed tomography

Head computed tomography (CT) as applied to stroke has evolved and become absorbed into clinical practice without systematic evaluation. There is, however, no shortage of 'expert opinion' which generally supports a low-threshold clinical policy to scan (Royal College of Physicians, 1990; US National Stroke Association Consensus Statement, 1993; Lindley *et al*, 1995a), but controversy exists (Wardlaw and Allison, 1994). A policy of 'routine' head CT scanning is a rather intellectually lazy approach. It is better to understand the advantages and limitations (*Figure 3.2*) of the investigation and to adopt a system of intelligent clinical questioning pertinent to individual patients with suspected stroke. A useful framework provided by the King's Fund Forum (1988) in their consensus statement is given in *Table 3.4*.

In practice, the main clinical issue dealt with by a head CT scan is in the important distinction between cerebral infarction and haemorrhage. This allows rational and safer use of anticoagulation or antithrombotic treatments. Clinical scoring systems cannot reliably distinguish between the two pathologies (Weir *et al*, 1994).

Guideline 6 (level C)

Patients should have a head CT scan if there is uncertainty about the diagnosis of stroke or if anticoagulation or antiplatelet treatment is contemplated.

Head magnetic resonance imaging

To develop acute stroke treatments with the potential

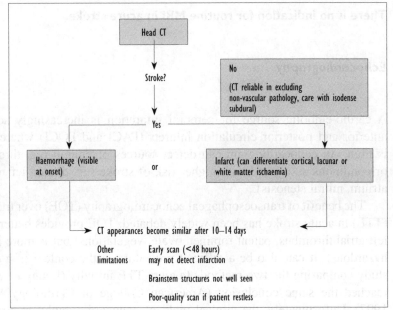

Figure 3.2: Contribution and limitations of head computed tomography (ICT) in acute stroke

Table 3.4: Framework for head computed tomography (CT) scan

Indication	Comment
Uncertain diagnosis of stroke	A head CT scan will reliably exclude non-vascular pathology. Care is needed to detect an isodense subdural haematoma
Current or contemplated antiplatelet or anticoagulation treatment	Main indication in practice
Suspected cerebellar haematoma	Potential neurosurgical intervention
Possible carotid endartectomy	To exclude haemorrhagic stroke and structural lesion mimicking stroke
Suspected subarachnoid haemorrhage	Potential neurosurgical intervention

to limit cerebral damage, the detection of early ischaemic changes seen on magnetic resonance imaging (MRI), but not by head CT has been considered an advantage. MRI is also able to demonstrate smaller lesions and image the posterior fossa, brainstem and lacunar lesions more clearly than CT. However, studies comparing CT and MRI provide unclear implications for clinical practice (Imakita *et al*, 1988; Mohr *et al*, 1995). Newer techniques such as diffusion-weighted MRI have promise (Lutsep *et al*, 1997) and may be incorporated into routine practice in the future.

Guideline 7 (level B)

There is no indication for routine MRI in acute stroke.

Echocardiography

A cardio-embolic source for cerebral infarction is increasingly sought, particularly in partial anterior and posterior circulation infarcts (PACI and POCI) where the risk of recurrent stroke is high. An echocardiogram can detect sources of emboli (eg. thrombus, myxoma, vegetation) or conditions associated with higher risk of stroke (eg. dilated left ventricle, AF and dilated left atrium, mitral stenosis).

The benefit of transoesophageal echocardiography (TOE) over transthoracic echocardiography (TTE) in acute stroke has been widely debated. TOE provides better anatomical information (eg. left atrial thrombus, patent foramen ovale, vegetations) but is more invasive (and therefore more hazardous). It can also be a difficult procedure in the context of a disabling stroke. The largest study comparing the two methods favours TTE initially (Leung *et al*, 1995) and a recent review reached the same conclusion (American College of Cardiology/American Heart Association, 1997). Unfortunately, the clinical yield of echocardiography in stroke is very low and routine echocardiography cannot be recommended (Leung *et al*, 1995; Chambers *et al*, 1997). It is more sensible to select patients for this investigation first, by whether a positive scan would change clinical management (usually initiation of anticoagulation), and second where clinical features or an abnormal ECG suggests cardiac disease.

Guideline 8 (level B)

There is no indication for routine echocardiogram in acute stroke.

Carotid duplex Doppler scan

A carotid duplex Doppler scan is a reliable non-invasive investigation for carotid artery stenosis provided it is performed by an experienced operator (Humphrey, 1995). There is good evidence that symptomatic patients with severe stenosis (about 80% or greater stenosis) benefit from endarterectomy by an experienced surgical team, whereas patients with moderate stenosis do not (North American Symptomatic Carotid Endarterectomy Trial Collaborators, 1991; European Carotid Surgery Trialists' Collaborative Group, 1998). Only patients with similar characteristics to those recruited to the RCTs and who are therefore suitable candidates for carotid endarterectomy should be investigated (Brown and Humphrey, 1992):

1. Patients with a minor ischaemic stroke in the carotid artery territory and little persisting disability.
2. Patients with a more substantial stroke in the carotid territory who have made a good recovery.
3. Patients who are otherwise medically fit.

Guideline 9 (level A)

Carotid duplex Doppler scan is indicated for selected patients only.

Management

General care and support

❖ **Fever:** The presence of fever in acute stroke is accompanied by a worse prognosis (Azzimondi *et al*, 1995; Reith *et al*, 1996). At present, it is not known whether the relationship is causal or a reflection of stroke severity. Obviously, a fever should prompt a search for an infection source. Antipyretics, although often used as a symptomatic treatment, are not known to influence outcome.

❖ **Hypoxia:** The level of oxygen saturation may be critical in the potentially salvageable ischaemic penumbra zone surrounding the area of neuronal death. Hypoxia is exacerbated by seizures, cardiac arrhythmia and pneumonia, all of which are associated with a worse cognitive outcome (Moroney *et al*, 1996). Correction of hypoxia seems sensible, although there is no evidence to suggest that outcome is improved.

Cerebral oxygen delivery might also be improved by haemodilution or by hyperbaric oxygen treatment. Haemodilution using venesection and/or plasma expanders aims to reduce haematocrit levels, thereby increasing cerebral blood flow but a systematic review shows no evidence for efficacy (Asplund *et al*, 1997). Hyperbaric oxygen is similarly ineffective (Anderson *et al*, 1991; Nighoghossian *et al*, 1995).

Guideline 10 (level B)

Arterial blood gases should be checked if hypoxia if suspected.

❖ **Cerebral oedema:** Therapeutic strategies to reduce cerebral oedema complicating acute stroke have been investigated but none have proved successful. Cerebral oedema related to tumours (vasogenic oedema) responds well to corticosteroids but cerebral oedema complicating acute stroke (cytotoxic oedema) does not. There is no effect on survival or improvement in functional outcome (Tellez and Bauer, 1973; Poungvarin *et al*, 1987; Qizilbash *et al*, 1997).

The two hyperosmolar agents, mannitol and glycerol, have also been evaluated but studies involving mannitol have largely been confined to the context of neurosurgery and animal models (Paczynski *et al*, 1997). A meta-analysis of RCTs investigating glycerol provides insufficient evidence to support its use, as, although there is a trend towards improved short-term outcome, the estimate of effect is statistically inconclusive (Rogvi-Hansen and Boysen, 1997).

Guideline 11 (level A)

Corticosteroids or hyperosmolar agents to reduce cerebral oedema in acute stroke are unproven treatments and should not be used.

❖ **Blood pressure:** Hypertensive encephalopathy and aortic dissection associated with hypertension may present with an acute stroke syndrome and both require urgent attention to BP control. However, for most patients with raised BP detected immediately after stroke onset, BP will fall spontaneously during the first tendays (Wallace and Levy, 1981; Morfis *et al*, 1997). This is a particularly vulnerable period as cerebrovascular autoregulation is impaired and injudicious reduction in BP might cause further damaging hypoperfusion in the ischaemic penumbra tissue. The converse, important clinical consideration is that low BP needs prompt correction of hypovolaemia and withdrawal of hypotensive medication.

There is unequivocal evidence for hypertension treatment in primary stroke prevention (Collins and MacMahon, 1994), but hypertension treatment in stroke survivors is much less clear and will remain so until the results of current RCTs in this area become available (Neal *et al*, 1996). Simple extrapolation from the primary prevention trials to stroke survivors is unwise as although patients have higher absolute risk of further vascular events and therefore greater potential benefit, BP reduction in patients with possible stenotic vascular segments may be harmful by inducing hypoperfusion events. Reassuring observational data were obtained from the UK TIA aspirin trial (1991) where a direct and continuous relationship was found between systolic and diastolic BP and further stroke such that a 5 mmHg reduction of diastolic BP was associated with about a third fewer recurrent strokes.

Guideline 12 (level B)

Record BP at least twice a day. Correct low BP where possible. Defer any reduction in acute BP for ten days unless hypertensive encephalopathy or aortic dissection is present.

❖ **Atrial fibrillation:** Patients presenting with an ischaemic stroke and non-rheumatic AF have a higher mortality (early and late) (Framingham Study, 1996) and are at high relative risk (12%) of a further stroke in the year after the event. The European Atrial Fibrillation Trial (EAFT, 1993) recruited patients presenting with TIA or minor ischaemic stroke within the previous three months and demonstrated that anticoagulation with warfarin reduced the risk of a further stroke by 67% and aspirin by 14%. Patients with major strokes (needing some assistance to walk and for personal care) were excluded. Major complicating bleeding events were low in the trialists' hands (warfarin 2.8%/year; aspirin 0.9%/year) probably because of careful patient selection and fastidious international normalised ratio (INR) control.

Thus, where there is no contraindication, and the patient consents, warfarin should be used for secondary prevention and, in other circumstances, aspirin. Subsequent work has indicated that the target INR should be 2–4: an INR of less than 2 has little treatment effect and greater than 5 carries a high risk of a bleeding complication (EAFT, 1995; Stroke Prevention in Atrial Fibrillation Investigators [SPAF] III, 1996). When to commence warfarin is not known, but waiting at least forty-eight hours, and possibly longer for larger infarcts, has been advised (Sherman *et al*, 1995).

Guideline 13 (level A/B)

Patients with AF and ischaemic stroke resulting in mild disability who have no anticoagulation contraindication should be treated with warfarin (INR 2–4) after waiting at least forty-eight hours. Aspirin should be used in other circumstances.

❖ **Blood glucose:** A glucose level greater than 8 mmol/litre is an independent predictor of poor outcome after acute stroke (Weir *et al*, 1997). The outcome of patients presenting with acute myocardial infarction and random blood sugars greater than 11 is improved by intensive insulin therapy (Malmberg *et al*, 1995, 1997), but it is not yet known whether a similar intensive approach to hyperglycaemia management in acute stroke is beneficial.

Guideline 14 (level B/C)

Measure blood sugar on admission for all patients. If high, or patient known to have diabetes, monitor blood sugars at six-hourly intervals.

* **Cholesterol:** Epidemiological studies do not support the notion of cholesterol as an independent risk factor for cerebrovascular disease (Prospective Studies Collaboration, 1995) and there are no intervention studies examining cholesterol lowering in patients presenting with stroke. However, a meta-analysis of trials investigating cholesterol reduction by a statin for patients with ischaemic heart disease has demonstrated an overall stroke risk reduction of 30% (Blaun *et al*, 1997; Herbert *et al*, 1997). Many patients presenting with stroke will have co-existing ischaemic heart disease and will therefore fulfil the entry criteria of these coronary secondary prevention trials. A reduction of baseline total cholesterol of 4.8 mmol/litre has been associated with benefit (Sacks *et al*, 1996).

Guideline 15 (level A)

Stroke survivors with a background of ischaemic heart disease and reasonable medium term prognosis (two to three years) with a cholesterol greater than 4.8 mmol/litre should be treated with a statin.

Prevention of early complications

* **Deep vein thrombosis:** Detailed studies have shown that deep vein thrombosis (DVT) complicates stroke in about 50% of patients during the first ten days (Kalra *et al*, 1995), but pulmonary embolus is much less common (6%–16% of patients; Sandercock *et al*, 1993). Although heparin, particularly low molecular weight heparin, is effective in preventing DVT complicating acute stroke (Sandercock *et al*, 1993; Counsell and Sandercock, 1997), the risk of haemorrhagic complications, particularly intracerebral haemorrhage, has been less well understood.

    The International Stroke Trial (IST, 1997) showed that subcutaneous heparin (12500 IU or 5000 IU twice daily) is associated with a significant excess of extracranial and intracranial haemorrhages and only a small and inconclusive reduction in pulmonary embolism confined to the higher dose heparin regimen, for which haemorrhagic complications were greater.

    Graduated compression stockings have proven benefit in the prevention of DVT in surgical patients but have not yet been evaluated in stroke (Clagett *et al*, 1992; Wells *et al*, 1994). They should not be used if peripheral arterial insufficiency exists as ischaemic skin damage may result.

Guideline 16 (level A/C)

Subcutaneous heparin to prevent DVT should be avoided. Graduated stockings are of uncertain effectiveness but should not be used in patients with concomitant peripheral vascular disease.

❖ **Pressure ulcers:** Pressure ulcers are a preventable early complication of an acute stroke which has resulted in immobility. Prevention involves assessment of risk and rapid deployment of special low-pressure mattress systems which are more effective than standard hospital mattresses (Effective Health Care, 1995).

Guideline 17 (level A/B)

Patients should be routinely assessed for pressure ulcer risk and those with high risk provided with a specialised pressure-lowering system.

Management of cerebral infarction

Occlusion of a cerebral artery results in a central area of severe focal ischaemia surrounded by an area of moderate ischaemia where the neuronal cell membrane is intact but the cell becomes electrically silent and synaptic transmission fails (ischaemic penumbra). A complex and incompletely understood process (Pusinelli, 1992) may further damage this area of relative ischaemia, extending the final infarct size. Pharmacological modification of the ischaemic penumbra process is an attractive goal but no drug has yet proved clinically successful (Langhorne and Stott, 1995). Modification of associated cerebral oedema has also been unsuccessful (see above). Only antithrombotics and anticoagulants are currently of proven benefit, in relation to prevention of further vascular events (secondary prevention) rather than direct acute infarct-modifying effects.

❖ **Anti-platelet therapy:** Aspirin is the most studied agent. A dose of 75–150 mg/day inhibits platelet cyclo-oxygenase and reduces the risk of further stroke and other vascular events by 22%, about forty vascular events avoided per 1000 patients treated over three years (Antiplatelet Trialist Collaboration, 1994). Larger doses of aspirin are no more effective but are associated with more side-effects, especially gastropathy (Weil *et al*, 1995).

Two large studies (CAST, 1997; IST, 1997) have shown additional benefit when aspirin is started within forty-eight hours of stroke onset (ten deaths or recurrent strokes per 1000 patients treated). Both studies committed patients to an early head CT scan to exclude intracerebral haemorrhage, when antiplatelet agents are contraindicated. Rapid onset of action requires a loading dose of at least 150 mg which can be given orally or rectally. Aspirin should be avoided if there is a history of aspirin hypersensitivity, active peptic ulcer or recent gastrointestinal bleeding, or if the patient is already taking an anticoagulant. The relative benefit of aspirin in each stroke sub-type (TACI,

PACI, LACI or POCI) is inconclusive (CAST, 1997; IST, 1997). This is not surprising as there is variation in the natural history of cerebrovascular disease: even when the first event is lacunar, further events may be embolic (Kappelle *et al*, 1995; Yamamoto and Bogousslavsky, 1998).

There is less information available for other antiplatelet drugs such as dypiridamole (Antiplatelets Trialist Collaboration, 1994), ticlopidine (Hass *et al*, 1989; Antiplatelets Trialist Collaboration, 1994) and clopidogrel (CAPRIE, 1996). They have similar efficacy to aspirin and can be used as (more expensive) alternatives. These agents have different modes of action to aspirin and therefore synergy is possible (Diener *et al*, 1996), but not yet well-established.

Guideline 18 (level A)

Aspirin should be given immediately in conscious patients with no contraindication provided a head CT scan result will be quickly available to exclude intracerebral haemorrhage.

❖ **Anticoagulant therapy:** *Warfarin*: The role of warfarin in stroke in the presence of AF is now well-defined (see above) but its use in the presence of sinus rhythm has been more uncertain. The Stroke Prevention in Reversible Ischaemia Trial (SPIRIT, 1997) compared low dose aspirin (30 mg) with warfarin (INR 3–4.5) in patients who had had TIA or minor stroke within the last six months and were in sinus rhythm. The trial was stopped early because of a significant excess of haemorrhagic complications in the warfarin group.

Heparin: The efficacy and safety of early anticoagulation was unclear until IST (1997) addressed this issue. Low dose heparin (5000 IU twice daily) was associated with a small but significant reduction in early death or stroke (twelve fewer events per 1000 patients treated) and a slight but non-significant excess of haemorrhagic complications. However, the observed treatment effect was no greater than that seen with aspirin. A medium-dose heparin regimen (12500 IU twice daily) had the same treatment benefit but with significantly greater hazard. In the sub-group of patients with AF, the balance of clinical benefit to hazard did not support the use of subcutaneous heparin.

Guideline 19 (level A)

Avoid subcutaneous heparin.

❖ **Thrombolysis:** One trial using tissue plasminogen activator in highly selected patients, in circumstances which would be difficult to replicate in routine practice, has reported a significant reduction in poor functional outcome (NINDS rt-PA Stroke Study, 1995). However, a systematic review and statistical summary of all available evidence indicates that considerable caution is needed. The meta-analysis findings (Wardlaw *et al*, 1997) show uncertain clinical benefit at the expense of greater hazard (increased symptomatic intracranial haemorrhage).

Guideline 19 (level A)

Avoid thrombolysis.

❖ **Treatment of cerebral haemorrhage:** The main initial management of cerebral haemorrhage is supportive care as outlined above. Surgical evacuation of a supratentorial intracerebral haemorrhage is controversial and probably best avoided (Hankey and Hon, 1997; Prasad and Shrivastava, 1997). Surgery for a infratentorial (cerebellar) haemorrhage is more widely accepted (Shenkin and Zavala, 1982; Hankey and Hon, 1997). The main indication is deteriorating or depressed conscious state.

Guideline 20 (level A)

Patients with a cerebellar haematoma and depressed conscious level should be referred urgently to a neurosurgeon.

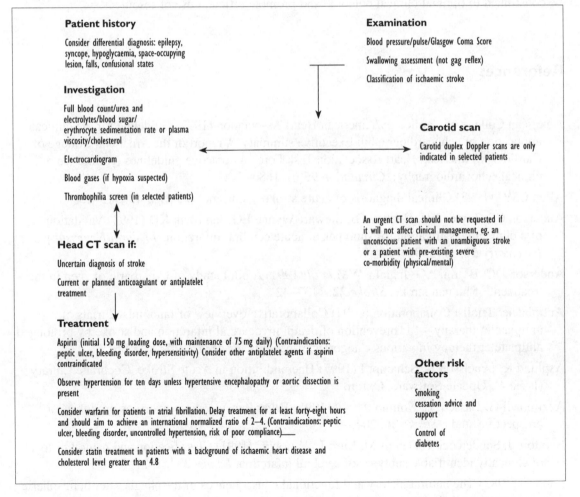

Patient history

Consider differential diagnosis: epilepsy, syncope, hypoglycaemia, space-occupying lesion, falls, confusional states

Investigation

Full blood count/urea and electrolytes/blood sugar/ erythrocyte sedimentation rate or plasma viscosity/cholesterol

Electrocardiogram

Blood gases (if hypoxia suspected)

Thrombophilia screen (in selected patients)

Head CT scan if:

Uncertain diagnosis of stroke

Current or planned anticoagulant or antiplatelet treatment

Treatment

Aspirin (initial 150 mg loading dose, with maintenance of 75 mg daily) (Contraindications: peptic ulcer, bleeding disorder, hypersensitivity) Consider other antiplatelet agents if aspirin contraindicated

Observe hypertension for ten days unless hypertensive encephalopathy or aortic dissection is present

Consider warfarin for patients in atrial fibrillation. Delay treatment for at least forty-eight hours and should aim to achieve an international normalized ratio of 2–4. (Contraindications: peptic ulcer, bleeding disorder, uncontrolled hypertension, risk of poor compliance)

Consider statin treatment in patients with a background of ischaemic heart disease and cholesterol level greater than 4.8

Examination

Blood pressure/pulse/Glasgow Coma Score

Swallowing assessment (not gag reflex)

Classification of ischaemic stroke

Carotid scan

Carotid duplex Doppler scans are only indicated in selected patients

An urgent CT scan should not be requested if it will not affect clinical management, eg. an unconscious patient with an unambiguous stroke or a patient with pre-existing severe co-morbidity (physical/mental)

Other risk factors

Smoking cessation advice and support

Control of diabetes

Figure 3.3: Summary of clinical guidelines for early management of stroke. CT = computed tomography

Conclusions

Clinical guidelines are 'systematically developed statements to assist practitioner and patient decisions about appropriate health care for specific clinical circumstances' (Field and Lohr, 1992). Guidelines have the capability to change clinical practice and affect patient outcomes (Effective Health Care, 1994). Stroke is a condition eminently suited to guideline-based management because it is common, has a widely dispersed evidence-base, and injudicious interventions readily contribute to a detrimental outcome.

These guidelines are based on desirable attributes (Effective Health Care, 1994), particularly a strong and explicitly linked relationship to the supportive evidence. The simplicity and clarity should maximise their implementation by the target audience: the admitting junior doctor. To further facilitate implementation, the guidelines are summarised in a simple flow diagram (*Figure 3.3*) which draws together the principle of structured assessment, careful individual patient-focused investigation, and considered treatment. In this way, an individualised care pathway can be constituted to optimal clinical outcome and promote efficient use of resources.

References

American College of Cardiology/American Heart Association (1997) Guideline for the clinical application of echocardiography: Executive summary. A report of the American College of Cardiology/American Heart Association Task Force on practice guidelines (committee on clinical echocardiography). *Circulation* **95**(6): 1686–744

Allen CMC (1993) Clinical diagnosis of acute stroke syndrome. *Q J Med* **43**: 515–23

Anderson CS, Taylor BU, Hankey GJ, Stewart-Wynne EG, Jamrozik KD (1994) Validation of a clinical classification for subtypes of acute cerebral infarction. *J Neurol Neurosurg Psychiatry* **57**: 1173–9

Anderson DC, Bottini AG, Jagiella WM *et al* (1991) A pilot study of hyperbaric oxygen in the treatment of human stroke. *Stroke* **22**: 1137–42

Antiplatelet Trialist Collaboration (1994) Collaborative overview of randomised trials of antiplatelet therapy — 1: prevention of death, myocardial infarction and stroke by prolonged antiplatelet therapy in various categories of patients. *Br Med J* **308**: 81–106

Asplund K, Israelsson K, Schampi I (1997) Haemodilution in Acute Stroke. Cochrane Library (Issue 4). Update Software, Oxford

Azzimondi G, Bassein L, Nonino F *et al* (1995) Fever in acute stroke worsens prognosis: a prospective study. *Stroke* **26**: 2040–3

Bamford J, Sanderock P, Dennis M, Burn J, Warlow C (1991) Classification and natural history of clinically identifiable subtypes of cerebral infarction. *Lancet* **337**: 1521–6

Barer D (1989) The natural history and functional consequences of dysphagia after hemispheric stroke. *J Neurol Neurosurg Psychiatry* **52**: 236–41

Bath P, Butterworth RJ, Soo J, Kerr JE (1996) The King's College Hospital acute stroke unit. *J R Coll Physicians London* **30**(1): 13–17

Blaun GJ, Lagaay AM, Smelt AHM, Westendrop RGJ (1997) Stroke, statins and cholesterol. A meta-analysis of randomised placebo controlled double blind trials with HMG-CoA reductase inhibitors. *Stroke* **28**: 946–50

Bonita R (1992) Epidemiology of stroke. *Lancet* **339**: 342–4

Brown M, Humphrey P (1992) Carotid endarterectomy: recommendations for investigation of TIA and ischaemic stroke. *Br Med J* **305**: 1071–4

CAPRIE Steering Committee (1996) A randomised, blinded trial of clopidogrel *vs* aspirin in patients at risk of ischaemic events (CAPRIE). *Lancet* **348**: 1329–39

CAST (Chinese Acute Stroke Trial) Collaborative Group (1997) CAST: randomised placebo-controlled trial of early aspirin use in 20,000 patients with acute ischaemic stroke. *Lancet* **349**: 1641–9

Chambers JB, de Belder MA, Moore D (1997) Echocardiography in stroke and TIA. *Heart* **78**(Suppl 1): 2–6

Clagett GP, Anderson Jr CFA, Levine MN, Salzman EW, Wheeler HB (1992) Prevention of venous thromboembolism. *Chest* **102**(4): Suppl 391S–407S

Collins MJ, Bakheit AMO (1997) Does pulse oximetry reliably detect aspiration in dysphagic stroke patients? *Stroke* **28**: 1773–5

Collins R, MacMahon S (1994) Blood pressure, antihypertensive drug treatment and the risks of stroke and of coronary heart disease. *Br Med Bull* **50**: 272–98

Counsell C, Sandercock PA (1997) LMWH/Heparinoids in acute stroke. Low molecular weight heparins or heparinoids compared to standard unfractioned heparin in acute ischaemic stroke: a systematic review of the randomised trials. Cochrane Library (Issue 4). Update Software, Oxford

Davenport RJ, Dennis MS, Warlow CP (1995) Improving the recording of the clinical assessment of stroke patients using a clerking pro forma. *Age Ageing* **24**: 43–8

Davies AE, Kidd D, Stone SP, MacMahon J (1995) Pharyngeal sensation and gag reflex in healthy subjects. *Lancet* **345**: 487–8

Diener H, Cunha L, Forbes C, Sivenius J, Smets P, Lowenthal (1996) European stroke prevention study 2. Dipyridamole and acetylsalicylic in the secondary prevention of stroke. *J Neurol Sci* **143**: 1–13

Ebrahim S (1990) *Clinical Epidemiology of Stroke*. Oxford University Press, Oxford

Effective Health Care (1994) *Implementing Clinical Practice Guidelines. No 8*. Nuffield Institute for Health, University of Leeds. NHS Centre for Reviews and Dissemination, University of York

Effective Health Care (1995) *The Prevention of Treatment of Pressure Sores 2: No 1*. Nuffield Institute for Health, University of Leeds. NHS Centre for Reviews and Dissemination, University of York

European Atrial Fibrillation Trial Study Group (1993) Secondary prevention in non-rheumatic atrial fibrillation after transient ischaemic attack or minor stroke. *Lancet* **342**: 1255–62

European Atrial Fibrillation Trial Study Group (1995) Optimal oral anticoagulation therapy in patients with non-rheumatic atrial fibrillation and recent cerebral ischaemia. *N Engl J Med* **333**: 5–10

European Carotid Surgery Trialists Collaborative Group (1998) Randomised trial of endarterectomy for recently symptomatic carotid stenosis: final results of the MRC European Carotid Surgery Trial (ECST). *Lancet* **351**: 1379–87

Field MJ, Lohr KN (1992) *Institute for Medicine. Guidelines for Clinical Practice. From Development to Use*. National Academy Press, Washington DC

Framingham Study (1996) Stroke severity in atrial fibrillation. *Stroke* **27**: 1760–4

Grimshaw JM, Russell IT (1993) Effect of clinical guidelines on medical practice: a systematic review of rigorous evaluations. *Lancet* **342**: 1317–22

Hankey GJ, Hon C (1997) Surgery for primary intracerebral hemorrhage: is it safe and effective? A systematic review of case series and randomized trials. *Stroke* **28**: 2126–32

Hass WK, Easton JD, Adams HP *et al* for the ticlopidine aspirin stroke study group (1989) A randomised trial comparing ticlopidine hydrochloride with aspirin for the prevention of stroke in high risk patients. *N Engl J Med* **321**: 501–7

Herbert PR, Gaziano JM, Chan KS, Hennekens CH (1997) Cholesterol lowering with statin drugs, risk of stroke, and total mortality. *JAMA* **278**: 313–21

Horner J, Massey E, Riski J, Lathrop D, Chase K (1988) Aspiration following stroke: clinical correlates and outcome. *Neurology* **38**: 1359–62

Humphrey PRD (1995) Management of transient ischaemic attack and stroke. *Postgrad Med J* **71**: 577–84

Imakita S, Nishimura T, Yamada N *et al* (1988) Magnetic resonance imaging of cerebral infarction: time course of Gd DTPA enhancement and CT comparison. *Neuroradiology* **30**: 372–8

International Stroke Trial Collaborative Group (1997) The International Stroke Trial (IST): a randomised trial of aspirin, subcutaneous heparin, both or neither among 19435 patients with acute ischaemic stroke. *Lancet* **349**: 1568–81

Kalra L, Yu G, Wilson K, Roots P (1995) Medical complications during stroke rehabilitation. *Stroke* **26**: 990–4

Kappelle LJ, Latum JC van, Swieten JC van *et al*, for the Dutch TIA Trial Study Group (1995) Recurrent stroke after transient ischaemic or minor ischaemic stroke: does the distinction between small and large vessel disease remain true to type? *J Neurol Neurosurg Psychiatry* **59**: 127–31

Kidd D, Lawson J, Nesbitt R, MacMahon J (1993) Aspiration in acute stroke: a clinical study with videofluroscopy. *Q J Med* **86**: 825–9

King's Fund Forum (1988) Treatment of stroke. *Br Med J* **297**: 126–8

Langhorne P, Stott D (1995) Acute cerebral infarction: optimal management in older patients. *Drugs Aging* **6**: 445–55

Leung DY, Black IW, Cranney GB *et al* (1995) Selection of patients for transoesophageal echocardiography after stroke and systemic embolic events. Role of transthoracic echocardiography. *Stroke* **26**: 1820–4

Lindley RJ, Amayo EO, Marshall J, Dennis MS, Sandercock PAG, Warlow CP (1995a) Hospital services for patients with acute stroke in the United Kingdom: the Stroke Association survey of consultant opinion. *Age Ageing* **24**: 525–32

Lindley RJ, Amayo EO, Marshall J, Dennis MS, Sandercock PAG, Warlow CP (1995b) Acute stroke treatment in UK hospitals. *J R Coll Physicians Lond 29*: 479–84

Lutsep HL, Albers GW, DeCrespigny A, Kamat GN, Marks MP, Moseley ME (1997) Clinical utility of diffusion-weighted magnetic resonance imaging in the assessment of ischaemic stroke. *Ann Neurol* **41**: 574–80

Mahoney FI, Barthel DW (1965) Functional evaluation: the Barthel Index. *Maryland State Med J* **14**: 61–5

Malmberg K for the DIGAMI study group (1997) Prospective randomised study of intensive insulin treatment on long term survival after acute myocardial infarction in patients with diabetes mellitus. *Br Med J* **314**: 1512–5

Malmberg K, Ryden L, Efendic S *et al* (1995) Randomised trial of insulin-glucose infusion followed by subcutaneous insulin treatment in diabetic patients with acute myocardial infarction (DIGAMI Study): effects on mortality at 1 year. *J Am Coll Cardiol* **26**: 57–65

Martin PJ, Enevoldson TP, Humphrey PRD (1997) Causes of ischaemic stroke in the young. *Postgrad Med J* **73**: 8–16

Mohr JP, Biller J, Hilal SR *et al* (1995) Magnetic resonance *vs* computed tomographic imaging in acute stroke. *Stroke* **26**: 807–12

Morfis L, Schwartz RS, Poulos R, Howes LG (1997) Blood pressure changes in acute cerebral infarction and haemorrhage. *Stroke* **28**: 1401–5

Moroney JT, Bagiella E, Desmond DW, Paik MC, Stern Y, Tatemichi TK (1996) Risk factors for incident dementia after stroke. Role of hypoxia and ischaemic disorders. *Stroke* **27**: 1283–9

National Institute of Neurological Disorder and Stroke (NINDS) rt-PA Stroke Study Group (1995) Tissue plasminogen activator for acute ischaemic stroke. *N Engl J Med* **333**: 1581–7

Neal B, Anderson C, Chalmers J *et al* (1996) Blood pressure lowering in patients with cerebrovascular disease: results of the PROGRESS (Perindopril Protection Against Recurrent Stroke Study) pilot phase. *Clin Exp Pharmacol Physiol* **23**: 444–6

Nighoghossian N, Trouillas P, Adeleine P, Salford F (1995) Hyperbaric oxygen in the treatment of acute ischaemic stroke. A double blind pilot study. *Stroke* **26**: 1369–72

North American Symptomatic Carotid Endarterectomy Trial Collaborators (1991) Beneficial effects of carotid endarterectomy in symptomatic patients with high grade stenosis. *N Engl J Med* **325**: 445–53

Oxbury JM, Greennhail RCD, Grainger KMR (1975) Predicting outcome after stroke: acute stage after cerebral infarction. *Br Med J* **iii**: 125–7

Paczynski RP, He YY, Diringer MN, Hsu CY (1997) Multiple dose mannitol reduces brain water content in a rat model of cortical infarction. *Stroke* **28**: 1437–44

Pound P, Bury M, Gompertz P, Ebrahim S (1995) Stroke patients views on their admission to hospital. *Br Med J* **311**: 18–22

Poungvarin N, Bhoopat N, Viriyavejakul A *et al* (1987) Effects of dexamethasone in primary supratentorial intracerebral haemorrhage. *N Engl J Med* **316**: 1229–33

Prasad K, Shrivastava A (1997) Surgery for Intracerebral Haematoma. Surgical Treatment in Patients with Primary Supratentorial Intracerebral Haemorrhage. Cochrane Library (Issue 4). Update Software, Oxford

Prospective Studies Collaboration (1995) Cholesterol, diastolic blood pressure and stroke: 13 000 strokes in 450 000 people in 45 prospective cohorts. *Lancet* **346**: 1647–53

Pusinelli W (1992) Pathophysiology of acute ischaemic stroke. *Lancet* **339**: 533–6

Qizilbash N, Lewington SL, Lopez-Arrieta JM (1997) Corticosteroids following acute presumed ischaemic stroke. Cochrane Library (Issue 4). Update Software, Oxford

Reith J, Jorgensen HS, Pedersen PM *et al* (1996) Body temperature in acute stroke: relation to stroke severity, infarct size, mortality and outcome. *Lancet* **347**: 422–5

Rogvi-Hansen B, Boysen G (1997) Glycerol Treatment in Acute Ischaemic Stroke. Cochrane Library (Issue 4). Update Software, Oxford

Roper AH, Shafran B (1984) Brain oedema after stroke. Clinical syndrome and intracranial pressure. *Arch Neurol* **41**: 26–9

Roth EJ (1994) Heart disease in patients with stroke. Part II: impact and implications for rehabilitation. *Arch Phys Med Rehabil* **75**: 94–101

Royal College of Physicians (1990) *Stroke: Towards Better Management.* Royal College of Physicians, London

Royal College of Physicians (1994) *Stroke Audit Package.* Royal College of Physicians, London

Sacks FM, Pfeffer MA, Moye LA *et al* for the Cholesterol and Recurrent Events Trial Investigators (1996) The effect of pravastatin on coronary events after myocardial infarction in patients with average cholesterol levels. *N Engl J Med* **335**: 1001–9

Sagar G, Riley P, Vohrah A (1996) Is admission chest radiography of any clinical value in acute stroke patients? *Clin Radiol* **51**: 499–502

Sandercock P, Molyneux A, Warlow C (1985) Value of computed tomography in patients with stroke: Oxfordshire Community Stroke Project. *Br Med J* **290**: 193–7

Sandercock PA, Van Den Belt AG, Lindley RI, Slattery J (1993) Antithrombotic therapy in acute ischaemic stroke: an overview of the completed randomised trials. *J Neurol Neurosurg Psychiatry* **56**: 17–25

Schneider AP, Nelson DJ, Brown DD (1993) In hospital cardiopulmonary resuscitation (CPR): a 30 year review. *J Am Board Fam Pract* **6**: 91–101

Shenkin HA, Zavala H (1982) Cerebellar strokes: mortality, surgical indication and results of ventricular drainage. *Lancet* **ii**: 429–31

Sherman DG, Dyken ML Jr, Gent M, Harrison MJG, Hart RG, Mohr JP (1995) Antithrombotic therapy for cerebrovascular disorders: an update. *Chest* **108**(Suppl 14): 444S–56S

Smithard DG, O'Neil PA, Park C *et al* (1996) Complications and outcome after acute stroke. Does dysphagia matter? *Stroke* **27**: 1200–4

SPIRIT Study Group (1997) A randomised trial of anticoagulants *vs* aspirin after cerebral ischaemia of presumed arterial origin. *Ann Neurol* **42**: 857–65

Splaincard ML, Hutchins B, Sulton LD, Chaudhuri G (1988) Aspiration in rehabilitation patients: videofluroscopy vs bedside clinical assessment. *Arch Phys Med Rehabil* **69**: 637–40

Stroke Prevention In Atrial Fibrillation Investigators (1996) Adjusted dose warfarin *vs* low-intensity, fixed-dose warfarin plus aspirin for high-risk patients with atrial fibrillation: Stroke Prevention In Atrial Fibrillation (SPAF) 111. Randomised Clinical Trial. *Lancet* **348**: 633–8

Stroke Unit Triallists Collaboration (1997) Collaborative systematic review of the randomised trials of organised inpatient (stroke unit) care after stroke. *Br Med J* **314**: 1151–9

Tellez H, Bauer RB (1973) Dexamethasone as treatment in cerebrovascular disease 1. A controlled study in intracerebral haemorrhage. *Stroke* **4**: 541–6

UK-TIA Study Group (1991) The United Kingdom transient ischaemic attack (UK-TIA) aspirin trial: final results. *J Neurol Neurosurg Psychiatry* **54**: 1044–54

United States National Stroke Association Consensus Statement (1993) Stroke Clinical Updates IV(1): 1–12

Wallace JD, Levy LL (1981) Blood pressure after stroke. *JAMA* **246**: 2177–80

Wardlaw JM, Allison SP (1994) Controversies in management: is routine computed tomography in strokes unnecessary? *Br Med J* **309**: 1498–500

Wardlaw JM, Warlow CP, Counsell C (1997) Systematic review of evidence on thrombolytic therapy for acute ischaemic stroke. *Lancet* **350**: 607–14

Weil J, Colin-Jones D, Langman M, Lawson D *et al* (1995) Prophylactic aspirin and risk of peptic ulcer bleeding. *Br Med J* **310**: 827–30

Weir CJ, Murray GD, Adams FG, Muir KW, Grosset DG, Lees KR (1994) Poor accuracy of stroke scoring systems for differential clinical diagnosis of intracranial haemorrhage and infarction. *Lancet* **344**: 999–1002

Weir CJ, Murray GD, Dyker AG, Lees KR (1997) Is hyperglycaemia an independent predictor of poor outcome after stroke? Results of long term follow-up study. *Br Med J* **314**: 1303–6

Wells PS, Lensing AWA, Hirsh J (1994) Graduated compression stockings in the prevention of postoperative venous thromboembolism: a meta-analysis. *Arch Intern Med* **154**: 67–71

World Health Organization (WHO) MONICA Project Principal Investigators (1988) The World Health Organization MONICA Project (monitoring treands and determinants in cardiovascular disease): a major international collaboration. *J Clin Epidemiol* **41**: 105–41

Yamamoto H, Bogousslavsky J (1998) Mechanisms of second and further strokes. *J Neurol Neurosurg Psychiatry* **64**: 771–6

Zaidi NH, Smith HA, King SC, Park C, O'Neil PA, Connolly MJ (1995) Oxygen desaturation on swallowing as a potential marker of aspiration in acute stroke. *Age Ageing* **24**: 267–70

Stroke community rehabilitation: a classification of four different types of service

Joanna Geddes, M Anne Chamberlain

In the past two decades, a great variety of community rehabilitation projects and teams have been developed, which are not easy to classify. This study examined the usefulness of a proposed classification system for home-based rehabilitation services for people with stroke. It was descriptive, comparative and quantitative. Services were categorised into four types: early supported discharge rehabilitation; post-discharge community rehabilitation; GP-oriented community rehabilitation; and late community rehabilitation. The features of each are described. The rehabilitation of almost all (98%) of patients studied could be placed within these categories. Providers of services, such as primary care trusts, need to identify the needs of their service users and match them, if possible, to suitable provision.

In 1996, the Stroke Association launched a competition to identify and publicise good practice among community services that provided coordinated, multidisciplinary rehabilitation to people with stroke. The six finalists selected comprised five discrete multidisciplinary teams at Merton (south London), Worthing, Newcastle, Sheffield and Northern Ireland, and one service in Derby that was run by a coordinator who constructed temporary teams according to patients' needs from existing community therapists and personnel.

The finalists agreed to an independent evaluation over a period of five years. Previous publications by Geddes and Chamberlain (2001a, 2001b) have identified key aspects that help to ensure the smooth introduction and successful continuation of the rehabilitation teams and, following a descriptive, comparative quantitative study, these authors proposed a classification system for community rehabilitation (CR). The term 'community rehabilitation' is taken to mean rehabilitation that is provided outside hospital.

The purpose of this chapter is:

- To illustrate the various pathways to community rehabilitation that can be taken by patients following stroke.

- To test the usefulness of the proposed classification in differentiating between populations of patients receiving home-based community rehabilitation following stroke.
- To describe and compare the populations in terms of characteristics and outcomes.

The classification distinguishes four types of CR, determined by the time of intervention and source of patients. In this study, rehabilitation is overwhelmingly provided in the patient's home and a minority is seen in nursing homes.

Methods

Methods have been described elsewhere by Geddes and Chamberlain (2001a, 2001b). In brief, between 1997 and 1999, data comprising demographic details, duration of CR, levels of disability as described by Mahoney and Barthel (1965) at start and end of CR, cognitive and communication ability, outcome of CR and referrals to other services were obtained from 1073 patients receiving home-based rehabilitation after stroke. The authors analysed these data according to the four types of CR. *Table 4.1* shows how the four types were determined.

Early supported discharge CR refers to community rehabilitation provided by teams specifically organised to enable hospital patients to return home soon after stroke. Two teams (Newcastle and Sheffield, UK) were set up to provide early supported discharge, the former with ready access to home care provided by social services and to technical staff to fit rails and other small adaptations, and the latter with ready access to nursing support and equipment.

Post-discharge CR intervenes at the point of discharge to provide seamless care. In total, 66% of the patients treated by Merton and Northern Ireland, 39% of those in Worthing and 17% of patients in Derby were in this category.

GP-oriented CR treats patients who are not admitted to hospital. Almost one half (46%) of the patients treated by Derby, 25% of Worthing's, 15% of Merton's and 19% of Northern Ireland's patients fell into this category.

Late CR is provided months rather than weeks after stroke to patients previously admitted to hospital after stroke, referred by GPs or other community personnel as opposed to hospital personnel. Derby and Worthing treated the greatest proportions in this way (37% and 36%, respectively) and Merton and Northern Ireland the least (18% and 17%, respectively). In total,

Table 4.1: Allocation of patients to type of community rehabilitation

	Admitted to hospital after stroke		Referred by hospital personnel	
Type of community rehabilitation	Yes	No	Yes	No
ESD (Sheffield and Newcastle)	Yes	No	Yes	No
Post-discharge	Yes	No	Yes	No
GP-orientated	No	Yes	No	Yes
Late	Yes	No	No	Yes

ESD = early supported discharge

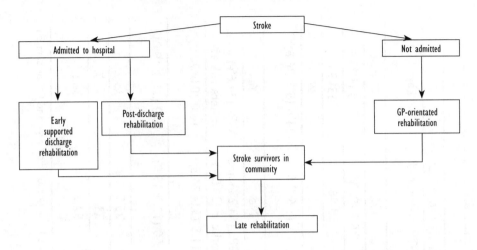

Figure 4.1: Pathways to community rehabilitation

87% of these patients had already received some inpatient rehabilitation. *Figure 4.1* illustrates the pathways to CR taken by these four populations.

One-way analysis of variance was used to examine differences between groups. The different types of CR were then grouped into early supported discharge and other types. A binary logistic regression analysis was undertaken to examine the characteristics of early supported discharge *vs* other types of CR. Where analysis involved a number of statistical tests across groups, the significance level (*P*) was set at less than 0.01.

Results

Data on 1073 patients who began a period of community rehabilitation between mid-1997 and mid-1999 were available for analysis. A total of twenty-three patients (2.2%) did not fit into the above classification system. They comprised four patients treated by Sheffield (providing early supported discharge) of which three were referred by GPs and one by another hospital, and the remaining nineteen were not admitted to hospital but referred by hospital personnel. The data did not allow clarification of these atypical pathways, hence they are not included in the analysis. The characteristics of the populations treated by the four types of CR and duration of CR are shown in *Table 4.2*.

Barthel scores are shown as the median (25th and 75th percentiles) since these are nonparametric data. Length of community rehabilitation is shown in the same way because of the uneven distribution of the data (the mean may give a false impression). *Table 4.2* shows that:

- The population receiving early supported discharge had the lowest levels of cognitive and communication problems, the highest levels of physical disability and the shortest duration of CR.

Table 4.2: Population characteristics by type of community rehabilitation (CR)

Characteristics	Type of community rehabilitation			
	Early supported discharge	Post-discharge	GP-orientated	Late
Number	318	311	190	231
Mean age in years (standard deviation)	68.3 (12.2)	69.6 (12.8)	76.1 (9.7)*	72.8 (10.7)*
Age range in years	27–95	29–96	38–96	33–94
Percentage who are male	51.4	49.0	43.7	48.1
Weeks since stroke (median 25th; 75th percentiles)	3.1 (1.7; 6.1)	9.4 (4.6; 18.7)**	3.1 (1.6; 9.6)	11.6 (5.9; 26.8)**
Admitted to hospital	Yes	Yes	No	Yes
Referred by	Hospital personnel	Hospital personnel	GPs (63.2%) and others (36.8%)	GPs (34.6%) and others (65.4%)
Weeks of CR (median 25th; 75th percentiles)	8.0 (4.0; 12.0)***	18.0 (9.0; 31.0)	11.5 (5.0; 24.3)	16.0 (8.0; 28.0)
Barthel Index score at start of CR (median 25th; 75th percentiles)	13.0 (10.0; 15.0)***	16.0 (11.0; 19.0)	17.0 (13.0; 19.0)	16.0 (11.0; 19.0)
Percentage with cognitive impairments	22.7	32.9	25.9	35.7
Percentage with functional communication problems	28.9	38.4	33.5	45.7
Percentage with **no** cognitive or communication problems	62.3	45.7	52.6	38.5

*Significantly different to early supported discharge and post-discharge CR (*P*<0.01); **significantly different to early supported discharge and GP-orientated CR (*P*<0.01); ***significantly different to post-discharge, GP-orientated and late CR (*P*<0.01)

- Levels of cognitive and communication problems were also low in the GP-oriented CR population compared with those of post-discharge and late CR populations. The majority of the GP-oriented CR population was seen soon after stroke (similar to supported discharge) but had lower levels of physical disability. The average age of patients in this group was significantly higher than that of those in the early supported discharge CR group. Almost two thirds (63.2%) were referred by GPs and the remainder by others, namely community-based therapists, district nurses, social workers, health visitors, Stroke Association family support workers, carers associations, carers and patients themselves.

- The post-discharge CR population was significantly younger than the GP-oriented or late CR populations but had relatively high levels of cognitive and communication problems.

- The late CR population had the highest levels of cognitive and communication problems and was the oldest population. Patients were seen on average almost three months after stroke; 65.4% were referred by others and 34.6% by GPs.

The data were examined by logistic regression, age and Barthel Index scores being dichotomised (divided into two parts) at the median. The analysis shows that, compared with all other groups, the early supported discharge population was 5.8 times as likely (range = 4.1–8.1) to start CR within six weeks of stroke; 3.5 times as likely (range = 2.5–4.8) to have a Barthel score below 15 at the start of CR; 2.3 times as likely (range = 1.7–3.2) to be aged seventy-two years or less, and 2.1 times as likely (range = 1.5–2.9) to have no cognitive or communication deficits.

These observations make clinical sense. It is more likely that patients willing to receive early supported discharge are on average younger, since they and their carers are less likely to experience morbidities associated with age. Carers would thus be more able to provide appropriate home support. Comparatively low levels (38%) of cognitive and communication problems would also be expected in this population, which must be able to cope after an early discharge from hospital.

It might also be expected that those not admitted to hospital would on average have less severe strokes. This is shown by the higher levels of ability (higher Barthel scores) at the same median time post-stroke as the early supported discharge patients. Cognitive and communication problems are also relatively less prevalent in this GP-oriented population.

The late population has the highest levels of cognitive and communication problems (61%), which is probably an important factor in their referral. *Table 4.3* shows the outcome at the end of CR for the four populations.

Patients receiving early supported discharge CR are most likely to remain at home and those receiving late CR are least likely. Early supported discharge patients showed the largest improvement in physical ability during CR. Selection of these patients for early discharge probably results in a population that is likely to make good progress. Those receiving late CR are accepted in response to need, with little selection. Their high levels of cognitive and communication problems will also affect their progress.

The increasing proportions of deaths and discharges to long-term care from early supported discharge, post-discharge and GP-oriented CR to late CR are almost certainly a result of the case-mixes of the four populations rather than any inherent difference in input given by the four types.

Table 4.3: Outcome by type of community rehabilitation

		Type of community rehabilitation			
		Early supported discharge	Post-discharge	GP-orientated	Late
Barthel Index score (median 25th; 75th percentiles)	Start of rehabilitation	13.0 (10.0; 15.0)	16.0 (11.0; 19.0)	17.0 (13.0; 19.0)	16.0 (11.0; 19.0)
	End of rehabilitation	18.0 (15.6; 20.0)	18.0 (14.0; 20.0)	18.0 (15.0; 20.0)	17.0 (12.0; 19.0)
Percentage outcome (*n*)	At home	94.0 (299.0)	86.2 (268.0)	80.0 (152.0)	72.7 (168.0)
	In hospital	1.9 (6.0)	0.6 (2.0)	0.5 (1.0)	0.0 (0.0)
	In long-term care	1.9 (6.0)	8.0 (25.0)	7.9 (15.0)	13.4 (31.0)
	Deceased	1.3 (4.0)	3.5 (11.0)	7.9 (15.0)	9.5 (22.0)
Missing data		0.9 (3.0)	1.6 (5.0)	3.7 (7.0)	3.3 (10.0)
Total no. patients		318	311	190	231

Transfer of care after community rehabilitation

Community rehabilitation teams do not exist in isolation; they provide a link in the chain of patient care and treatment, receiving patients from acute care, primary care or the community, providing rehabilitation, then transferring the care of these patients to appropriate agencies and individuals.

Just over half (54.5%) of patients who remained at home after CR were transferred to other services, as were 18% of patients who were discharged to long-term care. For those remaining at home, referral to other services was statistically significantly associated with levels of disability, whether physical (Mann Whitney P <0.01), cognitive or communicative (χ^2 analysis P <0.01).

Table 4.4 shows the numbers and percentages of patients referred to various services at the end of CR. Numbers add up to more than the total number referred since some patients were referred to more than one service. *Table 4.4* excludes those in hospital or in long-term care at the end of CR. No data were collected by Derby. The numbers who were referred to various services will have been partly influenced by the services that actually existed. The authors have no systematic knowledge to compare availability.

Referrals for further rehabilitation in the early supported discharge CR group include those to an assessment and rehabilitation centre by the Sheffield team and those referred for single therapy to community physiotherapists, occupational therapists, and speech and language therapists.

Social support includes carer support groups, referrals to social services, home care and social workers. Mental health includes referrals to psychologists, psychiatrists and community psychiatric nurses. Specialist clinics include neurological clinics, botulinum toxin clinics (for treatment of spasticity) and ophthalmology. Specialist nurses include diabetic and continence nurses. Miscellaneous includes mobility centres, chiropody, dieticians, wheelchair services, disabled advice officers and the Stroke Association. Patients receiving GP-oriented rehabilitation seemed least likely to be referred on to other services.

Table 4.4: Referrals by type of community rehabilitation

		Type of community rehabilitation			
		Early supported discharge	Post-discharge	GP-orientated	Late
No. in total population		305	280	129	173
Referred to:	Further rehabilitation	114 (38.1)	50 (19.6)	6 (5.3)	21 (14.8)
	District nurse	69 (23.1)	57 (22.4)	21 (18.4)	34 (23.9)
	Social support / social services	69 (23.1)	66 (25.9)	18 (15.8)	37 (26.1)
	Mental health	11 (3.7)	11 (4.3)	6 (5.3)	5 (3.5)
	Specialist clinic / nurse	13 (4.3)	7 (2.7)	1 (0.9)	2 (1.4)
	Miscellaneous	1 (0.3)	10 (3.9)	1 (0.9)	5 (3.5)
Total number referred on (%)		168 (56.2)	138 (54.1)	41 (35.0)	74 (52.1)

Discussion

In an editorial, Wade (2001) suggested various methods of classifying rehabilitation services and pointed out that the term 'community rehabilitation' has no accepted definition.

This study has been restricted to coordinated, multidisciplinary rehabilitation services for stroke patients, operating within patients' own homes or, for a small minority, nursing homes. Using the definitions suggested by Enderby and Wade (2001), five of the services would be described as 'client-group-specific community rehabilitation teams' and the sixth (Derby) as a 'community rehabilitation service organised by a rehabilitation coordinator'. The authors would describe the community rehabilitation provided as home-based, which gives patients access to interdisciplinary and interagency rehabilitation within their own homes and immediate environment. They would define it as 'multi-input home-based community rehabilitation'.

The authors' proposed classification system allows 98% of the patients studied to be placed according to the type of multi-input home-based community rehabilitation. However, GP-oriented CR should probably be split into GP-oriented early and GP-oriented late CR. While the median time after stroke in GP-oriented CR was roughly three weeks (early), a proportion of patients not admitted to hospital were referred by GPs months after their stroke (late). A weakness of the study is that the classification has been derived not from a general survey of community rehabilitation but from a selected group of CR services. It may be that other types of CR exist but have not been identified.

With this proviso, the authors suggest that the classification provides a useful guide when commissioners are deciding which type of CR could best serve their populations. How do these teams differ from intermediate care? The Health Service Circular to local authorities, which sets out guidance on the development of intermediate care services (Department of Health [DoH], 2001), expects intermediate care episodes to last no more than six weeks, apart from 'exceptional' cases (where patients may require intermediate care for slightly longer than six weeks). In this study, 74% of the patients received CR for longer than six weeks and the median length of CR was twelve weeks.

Intermediate care is intended for all diagnostic groups and there is a danger that the specialist skills needed for neurological rehabilitation would be wasted if teams were subsumed into intermediate care. Indeed, near the end of this study, one team (Merton) reported that, following a change in their management structure, the team was now part of intermediate care. The effects of change, they felt, included loss of team identity, dilution of specialist knowledge, lack of security and loss of direction.

References

Department of Health (DoH) (2001) *Health Service Circular 2001/01: Local Authority Circular 1. Intermediate Care*. DoH, London

Enderby P, Wade DT (2001) Community rehabilitation in the United Kingdom. *Clin Rehabil* **15:** 577–81

Geddes JML, Chamberlain MA (2001a) Improving community rehabilitation teams for people with stroke. *Br J Ther Rehabil* **8**(3): 92–5

Geddes JML, Chamberlain MA (2001b) Home-based rehabilitation for people with stroke: a comparative study of six community services providing coordinated multidisciplinary treatment. *Clin Rehabil* **15:** 589–99

Mahoney FI, Barthel DW (1965) Functional evaluation: the Barthel Index. *Maryland State Med J* **14:** 61–5

Wade DT (2001) Community rehabilitation. *Clin Rehabil* **15:** 575

Commentary I

The development of a taxonomy for stroke patients receiving home-based rehabilitation services is an important first step in matching identified service needs with service provision. Classification of the needs of stroke patients is particularly challenging because impairments can be cognitive, functional, communication, motor or, most commonly, a combination of the above and community rehabilitation (CR) needs vary widely as a result.

One of the more appealing aspects of this taxonomy is that it requires no sophisticated software and would not represent a significant cost to the user. Some collection of data is necessary, but this is already a quality-assurance requirement for many programmes and desirable for the tracking of patient outcomes. The classification is based only on a few key factors, such as hospitalisation, length of time since stroke, and the basis of referral. Moreover, while the authors admit that their taxonomy has not been derived from a general survey of CR but from a select group of CR services, this may in fact be an advantage. The select group of service providers included those who were most effective at providing coordinated, multidisciplinary rehabilitation services to stroke patients.

Although 98% of patients could be classified by this taxonomy, further refinement will be needed. Those referred by the GPs are likely to represent the most diverse group and, as the authors point out, may benefit from being divided into an early and late referral group. The late referral group may, in that case, not be all that different from those who were simply late referrals from a variety of other sources. Other types of CR (not represented in this study) may exist. Moreover, some patients could not be classified and this subgroup may need to be examined within the context of a larger sample size. Services and resources used within each of the groups will also need to be assessed and further subgroups may be defined as a result. Regional variation in availability of services will also play an important role in a final taxonomy.

However, this is an important first step, with the potential for allowing service providers and policy makers to identify needs and match them with available services on the basis of existing data. Although the authors chose to compare their early supported discharge group with the other three groups combined, this methodology would also allow researchers to compare the characteristics of the late CR group with the other groups. This is particularly relevant as it will allow healthcare providers and researchers to identify the characteristics of the population at greater risk for poor outcomes, allowing them to target those patients for additional services earlier in their course of treatment if appropriate.

In short, this relatively simple taxonomy may have important implications for the planning and provision of rehabilitation services for post-stroke patients within the community, and may be applicable to other diagnoses as well. It is hoped that additional research will provide important insights into the application of this taxonomy, both within the stroke community and beyond.

Wilma Hopman
Research Facilitator
Clinical Research Unit
Kingston General Hospital
Ontario
Canada K7L 2V7

Commentary 2

Hospital-based care currently dominates the management of stroke. Stroke units have received special attention — patients managed in these units are more likely to survive, regain independence and return home. However, it is concerning that this acute care model may become regarded as the solution to the management of stroke.

The 'inpatient approach' is highly developed in Germany and Austria. In these countries, after a few days of treatment at stroke units, patients are transferred to rehabilitation centres for a couple of weeks. Whereas stroke units and stroke rehabilitation centres cover almost the first twelve weeks after onset of stroke, nearly no structured community services for outpatients exist in Austria that provide coordinated multidisciplinary rehabilitation to people with stroke.

This British study demonstrates very nicely four different types of community rehabilitation (outside of the hospital) for stroke patients. The four types described cover nearly all patients who have to be treated in an outpatient rehabilitation setting and provide models for the implementation of such services in other countries. To my knowledge, few European countries have such a structured stroke outpatient rehabilitation programme as is provided in Great Britain. In view of significant differences in the healthcare systems of European nations, it would be a great challenge to implement the British model in other countries. This would be possible by modifying the national characteristics and deviations related to the British healthcare system.

The presented data indicate that a community-based stroke rehabilitation service works in different settings and is effective, given the huge cost of managing stroke patients in both financial and social terms. This study is also of high value since this concept can be extrapolated to the whole field of neurorehabilitation with diagnosis of, for example, brain trauma, multiple sclerosis and Parkinson's disease.

It is clearly recognised that stroke rehabilitation and neurorehabilitation require a longer-term perspective — probably at least three to five years after the initial stroke. There are obvious parallels with other chronic diseases. We have to argue for a more comprehensive rehabilitation approach, especially with greater emphasis on psychosocial functioning. This might be started in hospital, but its full realisation requires a community orientation.

Considering the efficacy of both stroke units and outpatient rehabilitation programmes, it becomes evident that both hospital and community services are needed. The effective delivery of post-stroke rehabilitation requires development of an integrated care system that spans acute care, acute rehabilitation, subacute rehabilitation, outpatient services, home care and community support services. Important developments for this are the use of clinical pathways, effective information systems, and communication between levels and sites of care.

Franz T Aichner
Professor of Neurology
Department of Neurology
Wagner-Jauregg Hospital Weg 15
A-4020 Linz
Austria

CHAPTER 5

Stroke rehabiliation: quality of care and levels of staff training

Yvonne Webb, Jo Pethybridge, Ruth Baker

A few weeks ago, I (YW) was admitted to my local hospital for some tests after suffering severe abdominal pain. The bed next to me was occupied by Edith, a seventy-one year-old former line-dancing, no-nonsense cockney, who, despite her poor health, maintained a cheery outlook on life, putting my annoyance at my (as it turned out, temporary) inconvenience to shame. Edith had received a hip replacement after a fall, but then had a stroke while in hospital. When I arrived, she was feeling much better, but her arm was weak, as well as her unoperated side. I marvelled at her good humour in the face of this double whammy. No doubt, a posse of relatives and friends who came to see her daily bolstered her resilience, but I had to admire her fortitude.

Edith told me that a physiotherapist had visited her a couple of times on the ward, and had told Edith that she needed to start walking, and to exercise her arm. The physio had promised to come back and help Edith to mobilise, but so far nothing had happened. Edith began to get desperate, wondering if she would be able to return to her previous independence and, most crucially, her line-dancing. Eventually, after chatting to her from my bed, I said loudly and in earshot of a passing nurse, 'You must walk, Edith — why don't you ask one of the nurses?' At this, the nurse came over and pulled a walking frame from the end of Edith's bed. 'Come on then, Edith,' she said. A moment later, Edith was shuffling with confidence to the toilet and back. Being heaved into bed, she smiled with satisfaction: 'I knew I could do it,' she said. Ten minutes later, the nurse returned. 'I've been told I should walk you regularly,' she said, hoisting out the frame once more. 'What, again?' asked Edith, incredulously. 'Yup,' said the nurse. Off they went, Edith beaming.

I relate this anecdote because it seems that, despite the considerable improvements in stroke care over the past few years, some basic rehabilitation procedures for stroke patients do not occur as part of routine practice. This might result from a range of variables that combine to get in the way, some of which include awareness of stroke and immediate post-stroke care among ward staff, which I will discuss in this chapter; others are more sociological and systemic, and may include communication and coordination between professionals, organisation structures and even general changes in society, such as the impact on health and social services of an ageing population and the decline of an available extended family to care for them. I have written elsewhere about the particular pressures on NHS staff caring for an increasingly elderly and frail patient population (there is a collective acknowledgement in my area, for instance, that the average age of patients has increased from sixty-five to over eighty years of age), which is more likely now to die in hospital than at home. These pressures weigh particularly on nurses, who often bear the brunt of the daily realities of hands-on care of increasingly frail patients with sensory impairment, incontinence, pressure sores and dementia (Webb *et al*, 2002), not to mention the degree of self-neglect, depression and generally poor conditions in which many have, somehow, managed in before being admitted. If stroke is not always treated as a priority, perhaps it is because it often comes with a whole raft of other problems — physical, psychological and social — which also have to be dealt with simultaneously.

This makes it even more important to raise awareness among staff working in all settings about stroke and its potentially devastating (yet often preventable) impact on all life areas for the patient. As I hope the following survey shows, many staff working with stroke patients do not have an adequate understanding of stroke and would welcome further training.

Background

In 2002, my colleague Jo Pethybridge and I were involved in carrying out a survey in stroke care services. All participating staff were those who provided care to stroke patients either on specialist units or on general wards. They were asked whether they had received training in the care of stroke patients and, if so, how adequate this training had been.

Half of the combined nursing and therapy staff working with stroke patients said that they had not received specific training, while the majority of nurses had received very little or no training at all, or the training was inadequate. In addition, we found that awareness of the specific needs of stroke patients was important among non-clinical staff, such as care assistants, ancillary workers and porters, who all play a key role in the course of patient rehabilitation.

Since our survey, there have been progressive improvements in stroke care services, with 85% of hospitals reported in the 2004 National Sentinel Audit of Stroke as having stroke unit. However, the audit team found that there continue to be wide variations in staffing levels between units and that, typically, only half of stroke patients will be located on a stroke ward, with the rest dispersed across general medical wards. Further, only 50% of hospitals reported access to specialist nursing support in stroke care from general wards, thus making continuity of care difficult, if not impossible, on wards where nurses had not received training in the care of stroke patients, and where stroke patients might not be viewed as a priority among a range with varying conditions.

The 2004 audit reports, 'Much of nursing care of stroke patients is delivered by care assistants'. Many of our findings, therefore, remain pertinent today, and suggest that more effort is needed in raising awareness, particularly among lower-grade nurses and non-clinical staff about the needs of stroke patients, as these will often be the ones with most patient contact. In addition, we found that nurses contribute less than other professions to multidisciplinary team meetings, and that provision of training and support to nurses to take a more active role in teamwork, and for others to recognise their input, is a neglected area.

Method

Seven hundred questionnaires were sent to therapy and nursing staff across seven NHS hospitals in north London, UK. The questionnaire items were based on the *National Clinical Guidelines for Stroke* (Royal College of Physicians, 1999), which provide a general standard for good-quality services, including areas of clinical care, initial assessment, rehabilitation, equipment, clinical records, support of relatives, communication with outside agencies, and discharge procedures. Staff members were also asked about staffing levels and about ancillary support for stroke care. Each item was rated according to a 4-point rating scale ('Excellent', 'Quite Good', 'Not Very Good', 'Poor'), with definitions for each quality rating.

Focus-group meetings and informal interviews were also carried out with small numbers of nurses and allied health staff in two hospitals.

Sample

Out of 700 questionnaires sent out, 157 nurses and eighty-seven therapy staff responded. Most respondents (88%) were female; 71% were under the age of forty years and came from a variety of ethnic backgrounds. They were thought likely to be representative of nursing and therapy staff working in inner-city hospitals. However, proportionally more therapy than nursing staff responded to the questionnaires, and the survey included only two doctors, as it proved difficult to get sufficient access to junior doctors because of rotations.

It is possible, however, that those who decided to respond were biased in one way or another in relation to the topic of the questionnaires. However, the experience of the researcher was that much depended on the willingness of senior personnel to encourage their staff to respond, rather than being a matter of self-selection.

Most of the eight hospitals had designated beds for stroke patients, and two had a specialist rehabilitation unit.

Results

Those who responded were generally positive about the quality of care for stroke patients in relation to clinical care (79%), initial assessment (85%), rehabilitation (80%), clinical records (79%), support of carers (78%), liaising with community agencies (79%) and discharge procedures (92%). They were less positive about available equipment, facilities and computer records. Overall, most thought that the quality of their service was 'Quite Good', although nearly a fifth thought that it was 'Not Very Good' and 3% that it was 'Poor' (*Table 5.1*).

There were considerable differences across settings (see below), different aspects of care and different professional points of view. The distinctions seemed to be mostly at the extremes of quality, as there was little disparity between the professions in whether the service was 'Not Very Good' or 'Quite Good', but there was a much larger discrepancy in whether they thought the service was 'Poor' or 'Excellent'. A fifth of nurses felt that the overall quality of care for stroke patients was 'Excellent' compared with only 7% of allied health professionals.

Trained staff (79%) were more likely to be positive about the quality of rehabilitation in their setting than non-trained staff (61%).

Those working exclusively on a specialist unit were much more likely to perceive their service as 'Excellent' compared with those working on non-specialist units (*Figure 5.1*). In other words, they perceived the quality of their service as

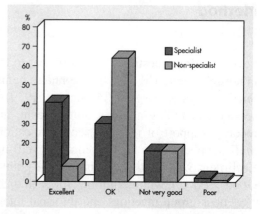

Figure 5.1: Perceptions of quality of care for stroke patients by staff in specialist and non-specialist settings

being extremely high across all aspects of care. Elderly and medical wards, on the other hand, were viewed as being 'Quite Good', but with limitations in certain aspects of clinical care and rehabilitation.

Table 5.1: Perceptions of quality of different aspects of care for stroke patients (n=244*)

	Excellent	Quite Good	Not Very Good	Poor
Clinical care	30 (13%)	154 (66%)	42 (18%)	7 (3%)
Initial assessment	59 (25%)	139 (60%)	34 (15%)	1 (1%)
Staffing	29 (12%)	122 (52%)	71 (30%)	14 (6%)
Support services	13 (13%)	142 (60%)	71 (30%)	10 (4%)
Rehabilitation	38 (17%)	138 (63%)	37 (17%)	5 (2%)
Equipment	50 (21%)	98 (42%)	69 (30%)	17 (7%)
Facilities	36 (16%)	108 (47%)	69 (30%)	17 (7%)
Clinical records	53 (23%)	130 (56%)	47 (20%)	4 (2%)
Computer records	17 (15%)	42 (38%)	33 (29%)	20 (18%)
Support carers	55 (23%)	130 (55%)	49 (21%)	4 (2%)
Community agencies	24 (10%)	159 (69%)	44 (19%)	4 (2%)
Discharge procedures	78 (34%)	134 (58%)	15 (7%)	4 (2%)
Overall quality	34 (15%)	146 (63%)	42 (19%)	6 (3%)

*Not all respondents answered all questions

Training

Staff participating in the study were asked how much training in stroke care they had received and whether they had an interest in stroke. Nearly half of the staff surveyed reported that they had not received specific training. Occupational therapists, speech therapists and physiotherapists working with stroke patients were most likely to have received specific training, while most nurses and nursing assistants reported having received very little or no training (*Figure 5.2*).

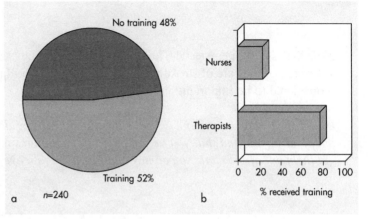

However, many allied health professionals, particularly occupational therapists and dietitians, felt that the training they had received was not

Figure 5.2: Proportion of staff (a) and proportion of nurses and therapists (b) who had received specific training in the care of stoke patients

adequate, while over half of the nurses who had received training felt it to be inadequate. Yet, all staff who had not received training cared for, on average, almost as many stroke patients per week as those who had received specialist training.

Of the therapists surveyed, occupational therapists, speech and language therapists and physiotherapists reported having received the most training. Dietitians had received less, but only four responded to the questionnaire, and it is unclear how representative they were.

Even in specialist units, training was often deficient. Of twenty-eight staff who worked only on a specialist unit, twelve said they had not received training, all of whom were nurses. This posed a particular problem for therapy staff working with patients dispersed across several wards:

> *There is very little carryover; the only way you get carryover is when you get to know a particular nurse and you semi-train her... and you look for certain things and make sure, for example, the [patient's] arm is not flaccid and hanging down by their side. But it is incredibly frustrating for us if these things are not carried over, as an hour in the gym or an hour dressing practice is wasted.*
>
> Physiotherapist

Many nurses were also aware of their lack of knowledge and training of how to position and care for stroke patients. They often felt unduly blamed by relatives and carers for deficiencies in care and services:

> *We need to assess more their [stroke patients'] level of deterioration, but I'm not confident enough to assess stroke patients on this ward.*
>
> Nurse on general elderly ward

Normally, you know what you are doing, but you don't know the extent of the care that you need to give. Sometimes the nurses turn the patient on the stroke side, which is supposed to be wrong. It is not clear. We have not had special training for this.

Nurse on general elderly ward

Nonetheless, most nurses who had no specialist training expressed an interest in learning more about stroke and the care of stroke patients. Training for ancillary, catering and domestic staff was also considered to be important:

Under the portering system, we have the patient coming down half an hour after they are due, and so you find that you've got only fifteen minutes left to treat them. You can't even get them out of the chair sometimes and just have to leave them sitting.

Physiotherapist in acute hospital

Patients were sometimes put at risk of aspiration because they had been given unthickened drinks or normal meals by catering staff who missed signs put up by speech and language therapists for soft-food-only diets and thickened drinks:

The problem is that for many [catering staff] English is not their first language, so they don't understand the signs by the bed. There needs to be more effort to educate catering and domestic staff in the dangers of giving patients normal food and drink when they cannot swallow it.

Therapist

Discussion

It may seem odd to ask staff to evaluate their own service, as it could seem that most will be biased in favour of the care they provide. However, the main reason was to establish whether there was an association between their perception of the quality of care in the setting in which they worked, and their satisfaction with, and commitment to, their job.

Clearly, the quality of care provided, and therefore of staff, will depend in large part on their technical ability and skills. Yet, only half of the staff surveyed reported that they had received training in the care of stroke patients. Many were keen, however, to learn more about stroke and stroke care. In the wider remit of the project, it was also found that staff who felt that they had had sufficient access to career development and training opportunities were also more satisfied with their jobs; thus, quality of care, training and job satisfaction were interrelated (Webb *et al*, 2002).

For nurses and therapists who are keen to learn more skills around stroke care, mechanisms are needed that will free them for extra training and support. However, a common complaint in this study was, that while senior managers supported innovative training programmes, staff on the ground felt unable to attend them without full backing from their immediate supervisors because nursing shortages were a daily problem. It was also particularly difficult for allied health staff to take time out, as no-one else could stand in for them with their caseloads. In addition, while many therapists working in stroke services reported that they had received training, they felt that their continuing training needs were often overlooked in funding allocation, or that their full range of knowledge and skills was not utilised. Thus, for example, speech and language therapists might find themselves only carrying out swallowing assessments, whereas, clearly, many stroke patients experience speech difficulties and would benefit from retraining.

Some therapists took it upon themselves to improve their knowledge of, and skills in, stroke care. Those in one hospital, for example, put on a stroke training day for nurses. There were twenty places available, although only twelve nurses could attend. The training day was very successful, although it had been at huge cost to those organising it, who had to prepare in their own time and needed help with presentation methods. In the event, the researcher provided a session on how to use PowerPoint and present material.

As well as formal events, therefore, options for training staff on-site (on wards and units) are also important, as the former are often conducted away from the workplace in an artificial environment, and it is hard to transfer manual handling methods which are taught in the lecture theatre to work on the wards, where the availability of equipment (such as hoists) and staff determine everyday practice. It was found that a high proportion of staff participating in the wider survey complained of having to take time off for work-related illness and injuries (Webb *et al*, 2002). This problem cannot be underestimated, and tackling it is still an upward struggle when speed and convenience often take priority over correct procedure.

At the heart of training is the communication of information and knowledge. Many staff learn 'on the job' by watching and listening to other more senior and experienced staff. Good-quality care and effective team working is as much about proper observation of patients, and communication of information about them and about what is needed from each professional involved in their treatment, as is each team member having the right technical skills. Moreover, as well as an adequate understanding of the occurrence and process of stroke as a disease, good care requires also common awareness and clarity about the role of different staff members (which can be alarmingly spare, even in multidisciplinary teams). This also includes portering, domestic and catering staff. Interviews and focus groups with non-clinical staff in one of the seven hospitals surveyed here revealed, for instance, that they did not feel part of the ward team, and felt unconnected to ward life and communications between staff about patients. Many were moved around to different wards, and therefore missed out on an opportunity to get to know patients and staff. Clearly, better communication to non-clinical staff might have prevented some of the instances where food and drink were left for patients with swallowing difficulties. Without a general understanding and respect for the role, capabilities and boundaries of working of each professional or staff group involved with a patient, there is potential for fragmentation and lack of team working, which can lead to a drift away from the priority goals of the team and setting.

Further work in this study, which included observations of multidisciplinary teams providing stroke care, showed, for example, that some professionals contributed more to discussions and decisions about care than others, which meant that important information about individual patients, such as their continence at night and their psychological well-being, could get lost when decisions about discharge were made, with the result that some patients could end up back in hospital after only a few weeks.

There was often a lack of understanding about different professional roles and responsibilities and how these may be affected by decision-making. Education and training might include helping all staff develop confidence about discussing and sharing their knowledge of individual patients. This relates, in particular, to those who are close to patients but who are not used to discussing patients' needs in a team setting, such as assistant staff. Education and training might also include raising awareness of the toll on therapy and nursing staff of caring for patients who are chronically ill or disabled (Webb *et al*, 2002), and in providing optimal care while working with restricted resources. My experience, both as a patient and as a researcher, is that patients in their fear, confusion, frustration and helplessness can be verbally abusive of nursing staff, sometimes extending to racism in its ugliest forms. Perhaps it is not surprising that, in my wider consultancy work, some nurses have told me they find themselves retreating to the nursing station or detaching emotionally in order to avoid these attacks (which can also come from patients' relatives). Moreover, the effects of stroke may often be complicated by factors beyond the control of the health professional, such as social isolation, housing problems, financial difficulty, chronic disability and associated mental health and emotional issues. We found that many staff worried how stroke patients would cope in the community. Indeed, they would be justified in their concern, as community specialist stroke teams remain thin on the ground (National Sentinel Audit of Stroke, 2004).

The reasons for Edith not being walked sooner were not clear. Were the nurses aware they should be walking her? Were the physiotherapists too busy? Were there other, broader issues at play, such as problems with communication, coordination and team working between professionals? Either way, formal training on all wards and settings for stroke patients is crucial, but so too is consideration of the wider organisational and professional dynamics around care of older people.

Conclusion

In March 2001, the Department of Health (DoH) published the *National Service Framework for Older People*. Section five of this publication concerns the care of stroke patients. If the requirements of national standards and of this publication are to be met, then the issue of appropriate care and continuity of rehabilitation on the ward has to be addressed. As well as the installation of stroke units, the appropriate training of multidisciplinary teams of staff who care for stroke patients is crucial, as is the preparation of trained staff for the provision of specialist care settings. It is also fundamental to the morale and well-being of staff who care for stroke patients.

Thanks and acknowledgements to the North Central London Workforce Development Confederation for funding the project; to all of those who took part in the research; and to the steering group members for overseeing the project.

References

DoH (2001) *National Service Framework for Older People*. The Stationery Office, London

Hickey JV, Grotta JC (1999) What is the role of stroke units in overall care? *Dis Manage Health Outcomes* **6**(4): 193–202

Pound P (1999) Does patient satisfaction reflect differences in care received after stroke? *Stroke* **30**: 49–55

Intercollegiate Stroke Working Party (2004) *National Sentinel Stroke Audit*. Organisational audit 2004 (concise report)

Royal College of Physicians (1999) *National Clinical Guidelines for Stroke*. Available at www.rcplondon.ac.uk/pubs/books/stroke/ (last accessed June 2005)

Rudd AG, Irwin P, Rutledge Z, Lowe D, Wade D, Morris R, Pearson MG (1999) The national sentinel audit for stroke: a tool for raising standards of care. *J R Coll Physicians Lond* **33**(5): 460–4

Stroke Unit Trialists' Collaboration (2002) Organised inpatient (stroke unit) care for stroke (Cochrane Review). In: The Cochrane Library, Issue 1, Update Software, Oxford

Webb Y, Stearn A, Pethybridge J, Baker R, Maloney G (2002) Nursing the nurses. *Nurs Times* **98**(16): 36–7

CHAPTER 6

Community stroke rehabilitation: a model of good practice

Jane Greene

This chapter describes the development of an award-winning multidisciplinary rehabilitation service for stroke which includes carer support, health promotion and goal-setting as a foundation for therapy programmes. Analysis of the effective elements helps explain the reason for its success.

The Ulster Community and Hospitals Trust Community Stroke Team, the first of its kind in Ireland and one of only a few across the UK ,was established in 1995 following the trend towards community care options in the early 1990s (Department of Health and Social Services, 1990). The team was presented with a good practice award by the Stroke Association in 1996, Charter Mark in 1997 and 2000 and, in September 2004, was shortlisted for the local healthcare awards, Innovations in Stroke Care, and continues to develop innovative ways of delivering care.

The Trust covers a community population of roughly 140,000, over both urban and rural areas, and aims to offer early rehabilitation to suitable clients following stroke. Although accurate figures are not available, it is estimated that there will be 250 new incidents of stroke in the area per annum. Given that 20% of these will die (Warlow *et al*, 2001), and a small percentage will make a full recovery, the remainder will benefit from early intensive rehabilitation.

The current guidelines from the Royal College of Physicians advise that:

> *early hospital discharge (before the end of acute rehabilitation) should only be undertaken if there is a specialist stroke rehabilitation team in the community and if the patient is able to transfer safely from bed to chair*
>
> National Clinical Guidelines for Stroke
> (Second Edition) (2004: 77)

This does not explain, however, what comprises a stroke team. It is clear from the stroke unit trials that outcomes are better if patients are cared for in stroke units (Stroke Unit Triallists Collaboration, 1997; Edmans, 2001), but there is no real consensus regarding the composition of a stroke unit. It is thought that the crucial elements are that the staff are interested in and knowledgeable about stroke, and that the care is coordinated. But there is currently no standardised training across the UK.

Evidence is emerging which supports the benefits of community stroke rehabilitation (Rudd *et al*, 1997) and, following a randomised trial of community stroke rehabilitation in Belfast, Donnelly *et al* (2004) concluded that a mixed model of hospital and community-based rehabilitation would lead to greater choice and a shorter stay for less severely affected stroke patients.

Table 6.1: The composition of the stroke team

* Coordinator / superintendant 3 physiotherapist
* Senior 1 physiotherapist 0.5 WTE
* Senior 1 occupational therapist 0.5 WTE
* Speech and language therapist (grade 2)
* Social worker 0.5 WTE
* Community nurse (grade F) 0.5 WTE
* Rehabilitation assistant 1.5 WTE
* Team secretary (grade 3) 0.5 WTE

WTE = whole time equivalent

The team

Geddes and Chamberlain (2001) urge us to nurture our teams through realistic induction programmes and professional development. They explore the real concerns that practitioners have about going into people's homes and having to deal with the situation as a whole. When practicing within the protected confines of a hospital treatment session, aspects of stroke, such as depression, are not addressed. It is estimated that at least 25% of stroke patients will have depression (House *et al*, 2000), and this can impede progress.

The Ulster Community and Hospitals Trust Community Stroke Team (*Table 6.1*) has recognised the importance of offering counselling and carer support as an integral part of the rehabilitation programmes and, therefore, has a social worker as part of the team. The social worker offers bereavement counselling to clients and carers and facilitates a support group, PACT (Patients and Carers Together). Recognising that the effects of stroke for both patients and their families are traumatic, PACT offers a safe and friendly environment where people can share their experiences, socialise, offer support and develop new friendships. The group raises its own funds in order to provide transport, outings and overnight trips away. Links have been developed with the local Chest Heart and Stroke Association. The main focus of PACT is that life goes on and everyone is trying to move forward.

The need for support was recognised as long ago as 1894 by Florence Nightingale, who describes the needs of the invalid who believed:

what a convenience it would be, if there were any single person to whom he could speak simply and openly, without pulling the string of this showerbath of silly hopes and encouragements

Team roles have evolved in response to clients' and carers' needs. The rehabilitation assistants supervise and carry out delegated therapy programmes which cross the traditional professional boundaries: for example, client goals in relation to shopping, which may include issues surrounding mobility, memory, concentration, money-management, comprehension, manual dexterity, self-confidence, reading, communication and continence.

The team nurse targets health promotion and secondary prevention. The means and the timing of providing information for stroke clients and their carers has been identified as a problem area for a variety of reasons (Intercollegiate Working Party for Stroke, 1998; Rodgers *et al*, 2001). It is the responsibility of the nurse to ensure that both clients and carers understand their illness and that information is given in an appropriate format as an integral part

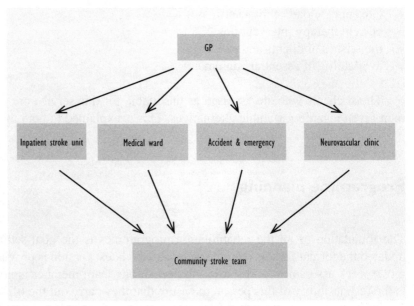

Figure 6.1: Referral pathway to the community stroke team

of the multidisciplinary care plan. Risk-factor management and health issues such as continence are assessed and appropriate management plans are put in place within the context of the patients' potential for recovery and their risk factors. Education for stroke patients and their families needs to be flexible and relevant to the person's abilities (Hanger and Wilkinson, 2001). The issue of primary prevention for stroke is addressed through opportunistic screening of family members, and onward referrals being made as required.

Eligibility/assessment process

The clients meeting the pre-set criteria are assessed following referral from the hospital stroke unit, medical wards or GPs (*Figure 6.1*). They need to be: medically stable; have a recent stroke confirmed with a computed tomography scan; have potential for rehabilitation; and have adequate support at home. The secondary care team will prepare assessments, the format of which was developed following a workshop with the stroke unit staff and the neighbouring community stroke team in East Belfast. The programmes are explained to the client and a family representative, if appropriate, in order to alleviate anxiety and answer any queries.

Following the publication of the Royal College of Physicians Guidelines (2000) and standard five of the *National Service Framework* (Department of Health [DoH], 2001), the team can highlight to general practitioners the benefits of referring patients with transient ischaemic attack or non-disabling stroke for secondary care assessment, either as an inpatient or at the fast-track neurovascular outpatient clinic. However, whereas the *National Service Framework* applies only to England and Wales, Northern Ireland would aspire to achieving the same standards.

Following assessment by the team coordinator, a discharge plan is developed, taking into account the following:

- current caseload of the team
- current therapy interventions
- the wishes of clients and carers
- availability of essential equipment.

Those clients who are assessed as unsuitable for this service are referred back and advice is then given regarding suitable alternatives. This is explained to both the client and the carer.

Programme planning

The foundation of all the rehabilitation programmes is the goal-setting process. The team has updated the format for this over the years and the latest version is proving easier to use. Following a two-week assessment and settling-in period, one team member is nominated as key worker. It is the responsibility of this person to ensure that they carry out the lifestyle questionnaire (*Figure 6.2*) with the social worker and, from that, help the client and his carer to set both short- and long-term goals. These goals are then brought to the rest of the team at the weekly clinical meeting, who will devise the therapy programmes around this. Each therapist helps the client to understand the use of specific techniques in relation to goal attainment, and target dates are then set. As goals are achieved, they are recorded in the client file, thus ensuring that the client and his or her carer can see that progress has been made. This is an important aid for motivation and can also be used to help both the team and clients to recognise when progress is not being made.

The programmes last for three to six months, depending on levels of need and how the clients and their families are coping. During the final part of the programme, the number of visits are reduced to help the clients move towards a planned discharge from the service. In order to reduce feelings of being let down, clients and carers can access telephone advice or reassessment of a particular problem. This 'letting go' phase has been identified as an unmet need and the team is currently devising an enablement programme to:

- facilitate coping and problem-solving
- alleviate anxiety
- enhance rehabilitation outcomes and social inclusion.

Every client is reassessed by the coordinator six months following discharge. The assessment includes a comparison of their level of disability with that at discharge, the mood of the client, health issues, socioeconomic issues and the carer's ability to cope. The coordinator is then in a position to refer the client and/or carer to statutory or voluntary community services, thus preventing further complications. The types of issues that arise are:

- splint repairs
- spasticity
- equipment for activities of daily living (ADL)

The following questionnaire is designed to help both you and your carer/family think about your lifestyle before your stroke and how things might have changed in your day-to-day routines.

We hope that you will have a clearer idea of your personal goals once you have thought about and completed the questionnaire.

<u>Guidelines on completing the questionnaire</u>

You will be given various lifestyle categories under each heading — we would like to give you some brief details under the three sections:

1. Before stroke — How important would this have been to you before your stroke? How involved would you have been in this activity and how often?
2. Now — How have things changed as a result of your stroke?
3. Future — What would be important for you to do again? Try to set some realistic targets to achieve.

Patient name: ....

Keyworker: ....

Date of completion: ....

Keyworker signature: ....

Client/carer signature: ....

<u>EXAMPLES</u>

	Before stroke	Now	Future expectations
Meal preparation	Prepared all meals.	Dependent on husband to do all cooking.	To make a cup of tea and light snack independently.
Housework	Husband did dishes, hoovering and fire. I did all other housework.	Husband and home-help do all cleaning.	To do housework only, eg. dusting.
Personal care	Shower or bath at least once daily. Hairdresser weekly. Make-up always.	Twice weekly bath at clinic — assistance needed with washing and drying.	Shower in own home daily with help. Weekly hairdressing. Help with make-up and dusting.
Personality	Outgoing, sociable, large circle of friends.	Low mood, emotional, withdrawn.	To enjoy interacting with people. To feel in control.
Mobility	Fully independent.	Wheelchair. Assistance needed with transfers.	Walk within home and to car (with aid if needed).

Figure 6.2: Personal home and lifestyle questionnaire

- driving/employment
- sexual difficulties
- depression
- carer strain/respite needs
- hemiplegic shoulder pain/central post-stroke pain
- incontinence
- hypertension
- medication confusion
- dysphagia.

It is noteworthy that both the Royal College of Physicians' guidelines (2004) and the *National Service Framework* (2001) highlight reassessment and long-term support as good practice.

As the clients are having a number of different professional staff coming into their homes, appointments are made using a client diary. This gives the family a chance to plan their day and the team an opportunity to make the best use of time. For example, if a client always goes to market on a Wednesday morning, this is regarded as rehabilitation because the client is resuming pre-stroke activities which will benefit the client more than a physiotherapy session on that particular day. Thus, no-one visits this person on a Wednesday morning. This also allows for client choice and some degree of control.

Similarly, the therapists must negotiate. If a client requires physiotherapy, occupational therapy and speech therapy, he will not be able to tolerate these sessions one after another. The flexibility that is built into the service allows for this as well as for joint treatment programmes. Between therapy visits, tasks or exercises are prescribed and these can be supervised by the rehabilitation assistants or the carers, or carried out by the clients themselves in response to identified need.

Record keeping is a critical part of care. With so many different professionals treating at the same time, it was decided from the outset to have a single, multidisciplinary client-held record. Client-held records were being used successfully in district nursing in the trust area at the time and great care was taken with these records. However, this was a change for the therapists and the social worker. The team members were involved in the design of the file and, following management theories of motivation through job enrichment and ownership, this proved to be very successful (Handy, 1993). The file is updated on a regular basis in response to client feedback and team members' ideas. Writing clinical records, with the knowledge that they will be read once you leave the house, ensures a reduction in the use of subjective reporting and jargon. It is noteworthy that none of the records have been lost since this process was introduced in 1995.

The file in the home contains information needed on a daily basis, such as care plans and progress notes and a second file containing demographic and assessment details is kept in the office and may be readily accessed by all staff as and when it is needed.

To foster multidisciplinary working and in keeping with the Royal College of Physicians' guidelines (2004), seminars are held every six weeks, and responsibility for coordinating these is rotated annually. The seminars are attended by both the qualified and unqualified staff and the topics are chosen by the team. In the past, these have included:

- sexuality and disability
- memory assessment tools
- communicating with aphasic adults
- shoulder care
- risk-factor management and secondary prevention
- disability employment services.

In addition to the meetings acting as a forum for communication within the team, it is essential to liaise with the rest of the primary healthcare team and voluntary sector. The team has established complementary working relationships with Northern Ireland Chest Heart and Stroke Association, Speechmatters and the local Citizens Advice Bureau, and it is happy to provide reports on behalf of the clients in relation to benefit claims, driving and major housing adaptation.

Quality

Health service users are aware of the focus on user consultation (Department of Health, Social Services and Public Safety, 2001), and this has been an ongoing process for the Stroke Team since 1996. Every client is asked to complete a satisfaction questionnaire following discharge, and these are analysed by the quality and audit department biannually. This is now normal practice and the team has found that service delivery is easier if you ask clients what they want. The client and carer comments have been overwhelming and one carer even responded by presenting the team with a watercolour painting of the team in action to mark his gratitude.

Other quality initiatives in place are multiprofessional standard setting (Ellis and Whittington, 1998), including an annual audit cycle, the results of which are published in the support group newsletter, *STRIKE*.

To ensure continuity of care from the acute stroke unit, a care pathway has been introduced. This has enhanced communication by ensuring that professional reports are available in a timely manner both on referral to the team, during the rehabilitation period and following discharge. Goal setting reviews and six-month follow-up are included in the pathway.

Owing to the number of queries from colleagues, clients and carers, the team has gathered a wealth of information in the form of books, journal articles, information leaflets, local contact numbers and website addresses, and is now regarded as a well-established local resource. The downside of this is that sourcing information for others is time-consuming and there is no extra staff time allocated to this. However, the advantage is that the team can help support the delivery of best practice by others and up-to-date information for clients and carers.

Conclusion

The success of a team such as this lies in the motivation and skills of the members, and the fact that there has been little or no staff changeover since 1995 has allowed for a sound knowledge-base to develop. The model of a single line of management is workable provided that interdisciplinary relationships are fostered and respected. The area of stroke care is also ideal for this type of approach because clients' and carers' needs cross traditional professional boundaries.

The scope for imaginative joint treatment sessions and the sharing of core skills is wide-ranging and challenging in the current climate of resource-driven healthcare delivery. While the publication of national guidelines and standards has helped to establish a clear evidence-base for practice, there is still a paucity of research in the area of stroke care, and in particular community stroke care and rehabilitation. It is therefore incumbent on us all to carry out good-quality research to inform our practice. As Neubauer (1998) puts it: 'If we always do what we always did, we'll always get what we always got.'

The Community Stroke Team was presented with a good practice award by the Stroke Association in 1996, the Charter Mark in 1997 and 2000, and was shortlisted for the Northern Ireland Healthcare Awards, Innovations in Stroke Care, 2004

References

DoH (2001) *National Service Framework for Older People*. DoH, London

Department of Health and Social Services (1990) *People First*. Department of Health and Social Services, Belfast

Department of Health, Social Services and Public Safety (2001) *Best Practice, Best Care: a Consultation Paper*. Department of Health, Social Services and Public Safety, Belfast

Donnelly M, Power M, Russell M, Fullerton K (2004) Randomized controlled trial of an early discharge rehabilitation service. The Belfast Community Stroke Trial. *Stroke* **35**: 127–33

Edmans J (2001) What makes stroke units effective? *Br J Ther Rehabil* **8**(2): 74–7

Ellis R, Whittington D (1998) *Quality Assurance in Social Care*. Arnold, London

Geddes J, Chamberlain A (2001) Improving community rehabilitation teams for people with stroke. *Br J Ther Rehabil* **8**(3): 92–5

Handy C (1993) *Understanding Organisations*. 4th edn. Penguin Books, Middlesex

Hanger H, Wilkinson T (2001) Stroke education: can we rise to the challenge? *Age Ageing* **30**: 113–4

House A, Hackey ML, Anderson CS (2000) *Effects of Antidepressants and Psychological Therapies for Reducing the Emotional Impact of Stroke. Consensus Conference on Stroke Treatment and Management, Vol 31 Iss 8*. Royal College of Physicians of Edinburgh, Edinburgh

Intercollegiate Working Party for Stroke (1998) *Stroke Rehabilitation, Patients' and Carers' Views*. Royal College of Physicians, London

Neubauer J (1998) Personal development: a lifelong journey. *Adv Pract Nurs* **3**(4): 1–9

Rodgers H, Band S, Curless R (2001) Inadequacies in the provision of information to stroke patients and their families. *Age Ageing* **30**: 129–33

Royal College of Physicians (2000) *National Clinical Guidelines for Stroke*. Royal College of Physicians, London

Rudd AG, Wolfe CD, Tilling K, Beech R (1997) Randomised controlled trial to evaluate early discharge scheme for patients with stroke. *Br Med J* **315**: 1039–44

Stroke Unit Triallists Collaboration (1997) Collaborative systematic review of the randomised trials of organised inpatient (stroke unit) care after stroke. *Br Med J* **314**: 1151–9

Wardlaw J (2001) *Stroke: a Practical Guide To Management. 2nd edn*. Blackwell Science, Oxford

Warlow CP, Dennis MS, Van Gijn J, Hankey GJ, Sandercock PAG, Bamford JM, Wardlaw J (2001) *Stroke: a Practical Guide To Management*. 2nd edn. Blackwell Science, Oxford

CHAPTER 7

What makes stroke units effective?

Judi Edmans

An observational study investigated the differences between a stroke unit and conventional rehabilitation wards. Differences included having established philosophies, policies and procedures that were applied by all disciplines, twenty-four hours per day, and having the multidisciplinary team ward-based.

In 1988, the King's Fund Consensus Conference (1988) stated: 'stroke services in the United Kingdom were generally haphazard and poorly tailored to the patients' needs' and suggested that stroke care should be more coordinated. Since then, research evidence has shown that stroke care on a stroke unit can save lives and is beneficial to stroke patients in terms of recovery (Langhorne *et al*, 1993). Stroke units were defined by Dennis and Langhorne (1994) as units where 'care is organised and coordinated by a multidisciplinary team of professional staff who are interested and knowledgeable about stroke'.

Many studies have demonstrated these beneficial effects of stroke units by comparing them with conventional rehabilitation wards (Garraway *et al*, 1980a, b; Smith *et al*, 1982; Stevens *et al*, 1984; Indredavik *et al*, 1991, 1997, 1998, 1999b; Kalra *et al*, 1993; Ronning and Guldvog, 1998a; Juby *et al*, 1996; Drummond *et al*, 1996; Lincoln *et al*, 1997).

A review of the literature which examined the effectiveness of stroke rehabilitation was carried out by Langhorne *et al* (1993), completing an overview of ten randomised-controlled trials which compared stroke patients on specialist units with those on general wards between 1962 and 1993. Findings showed that stroke specialist units reduced mortality, length of stay and the chance of living in an institution one year after a stroke and improved functional independence (Langhorne *et al*, 1993; Dennis and Langhorne, 1994).

The findings of Langhorne *et al* (1993) were corroborated by the Stroke Unit Triallists Collaboration (1997), which consisted of representatives from each of the trials included. The Stroke Unit Triallists Collaboration carried out a systematic review of nineteen randomised-controlled trials, which involved a total of 3249 stroke patients. Its objectives were to define the characteristics and determine the effectiveness of stroke unit care compared with conventional care. The distinctive aspects of the stroke unit care determined by the Stroke Unit Triallists Collaboration were also documented by Langhorne (1997). These were:

- coordinated and organised inpatient care with weekly meetings
- multidisciplinary team care involving medical, nursing and therapy staff
- programmes of education and training for staff, patients and carers
- involvement of carers in rehabilitation
- staff interest and expertise in stroke.

One of the randomised-controlled trials in the Stroke Unit Triallists Collaboration systematic review was that of Juby *et al* (1996), carried out on the Nottingham Stroke Unit. Juby *et al* compared stroke patients on the stroke unit with those on general medical and health care of the elderly wards, which included 315 patients admitted to hospital. The results showed a significant difference in personal activities of daily living (ADL) at three and six months, but not at twelve months, with the stroke unit patients being more independent. Stroke unit patients were also significantly more independent on extended ADL measures at six and twelve months. In terms of mood, there was no significant difference between groups at three and six months, but the stroke unit patients had a better mood at twelve months. There was a significant difference in adjustment at six months, with the stroke unit patients being able to cope better psychologically.

After further analysis of Juby *et al*'s study, Drummond *et al* (1996) completed a more detailed analysis of ADL ability. They concluded that stroke unit rehabilitation improved feeding, dressing and household abilities more than occurred following rehabilitation on conventional rehabilitation wards, whereas mobility improved equally in both settings. Drummond *et al* (1996) felt that these results were attributable to the policies and procedures adopted by the occupational therapists on the stroke unit, rather than just the occupational therapy intervention itself. This was because the nursing staff on the stroke unit had been trained by the occupational therapists to continue rehabilitation with patients, particularly in tasks such as feeding, dressing and kitchenwork. Other reasons given were that any aids required by patients at meal times were readily available on the stroke unit, and patients often went home at weekends and were encouraged to continue kitchen rehabilitation with relatives. In general, Drummond *et al* (1996) felt that there was more emphasis on functional ability on the stroke unit than on general medical wards, whereas mobility was seen as a priority on all wards.

Again, after further analysis of Juby *et al*'s study, Lincoln *et al* (1997) investigated the effect of perceptual assessment and treatment on the stroke unit compared with that provided on medical or health care of the elderly wards. The results indicated that there was no significant difference in perceptual ability between stroke patients on the stroke unit and general medical wards on entry to the trial, but that the stroke unit patients had significantly less perceptual impairment at all stages after stroke, ie. at three, six and twelve months. Perceptual ability was found to be a significant predictor of outcome 12 months after stroke. Lincoln *et al* (1997) suggested that these differences were attributable to the increased awareness and recognition of perceptual problems by staff on the stroke unit. They also suggested that stroke unit staff of all disciplines adjusted their treatment when perceptual problems were present and used general perceptual treatment strategies to reduce the effect of these perceptual problems.

Although the literature shows the effectiveness of various stroke units, there is little written evidence to show what actually constitutes a stroke unit in terms of the process of rehabilitation for the patients. Kalra and Eade (1995), Lincoln *et al* (1996), Ronning and Guldvog (1998b) and Indredavik *et al* (1999a) have tried to identify differences in aspects of care between the stroke units and conventional rehabilitation wards in their studies. However, these studies only investigated specific aspects of care and treatment, such as Barthel Index score, mortality, discharge destination, length of hospital stay, medication. These questions still remains unanswered:

- What does a stroke unit really consist of in terms of philosophies, care and treatment given to patients?
- How and why does a stroke unit differ from a general medical or health care of the elderly ward in order to be able to produce these beneficial effects?

Therefore, to try to answer these questions, the philosophies, policies and procedures used on the Nottingham Stroke Unit during the Juby *et al* study were examined and compared with those used on conventional rehabilitation wards. This observational study was carried out by an occupational therapist who worked on both the stroke unit and on conventional rehabilitation wards during the Juby *et al* study. The aim was to identify how and why this stroke unit differed from the general wards in the same hospital, which may have contributed to the conclusions made by Juby *et al* (1996), Drummond *et al* (1996) and Lincoln *et al* (1997).

The Nottingham Stroke Unit

The Nottingham Stroke Unit opened in 1983. At the time of Juby *et al*'s study, it was a fifteen-bedded inpatient unit, which accepted patients from general medical or health care of the elderly wards within the Nottingham Health District, but which did not take admissions directly from accident and emergency departments or the community. Patients could be male or female and ranged from twenty-one to over ninety years of age, with the average age of the patients being about sixty-five years. The average length of stay was six to seven weeks, and there was an annual throughput of about 120 patients, of whom about 80% were discharged to their own home (unpublished stroke unit annual statistics). There were written philosophies, policies and procedures for this stroke unit.

Philosophies

The stroke unit had a written philosophy, which was that it seeked to provide an effective and efficient multidisciplinary approach to rehabilitation. The aim was to enable patients to live independently in the community following discharge, with the best quality of life possible. Furthermore, a high level of professional competence in all aspects of care was aimed for, which included the psychological needs of the patient and his or her family. There was also a responsibility to teach other professionals all aspects of stroke care. Copies of the written philosophies were given to all staff of all disciplines during their orientation period on the stroke unit. There were no written philosophies on the conventional rehabilitation wards.

Policies

The major policies on the stroke unit included:

- Blanket referral for rehabilitation for all patients admitted to this stroke unit, ie. all patients were automatically referred for rehabilitation on admission to the stroke unit.
- A twenty-four-hour approach, where the same multidisciplinary approach was used consistently by all members of the multidisciplinary team throughout the whole day, ie. nurses can deliver the same level of care as occupational therapists.
- Staff training regarding all the philosophies, policies and procedures used on the stroke unit on induction; this training was ongoing, with weekly teaching sessions coordinated by the senior staff of the multidisciplinary team on the stroke unit, who also monitored the philosophies, policies and procedures informally.
- Policies regarding positioning, moving and handling, transfers, washing and dressing, dysphagia, continence, wheelchair use, home visits, self-medication, meal times, discharge planning, named nurse, health promotion and secondary prevention.
- Open visiting to enable more carer involvement.
- Carer involvement in rehabilitation, ie. carers were invited to join in any therapy sessions to get involved in any aspect of rehabilitation.

On the conventional rehabilitation wards with no written policies, patients were referred individually to each discipline and there was no twenty-four-hour approach, little staff training, no set policies or set visiting times, and little carer involvement in rehabilitation.

Procedures

The procedures of the stroke unit included:

- Rehabilitation primarily followed the normal movement concept (Bobath, 1976) but other theoretical models were considered where appropriate, eg. movement science (Carr and Shepherd, 1987), the Brunnstrom approach (Brunnstrom, 1970), proprioceptive neuromuscular facilitation (Knott and Voss, 1968), the Rood approach (Goff, 1969) and the Johnstone approach (Johnstone, 1980).
- Encouragement for patients to take responsibility for themselves where appropriate, ie. doing as much as possible for themselves, providing they use the correct movement patterns, and encouraging patients to make decisions for themselves.
- Set procedures regarding positioning, moving and handling, transfers, washing and dressing, meal times, continence, self-medication and discharge planning.
- All patients were encouraged to sit in a variety of chairs during the day rather than just in their wheelchair and, where appropriate, they were encouraged to stand regularly.
- All patients wore their own clothes and got dressed every day, including wearing shoes rather than slippers.

- All patients ate their meals in the dayroom rather than by their bed.
- Patients did not rest on their beds except when they went to bed at night.
- Involvement of relatives/carers throughout the rehabilitation process by all disciplines.
- All aids belonged to the stroke unit and were therefore available at all times.
- Multidisciplinary meetings were held regularly in the form of multidisciplinary handovers, case conferences and family case conferences, which included goal setting and care planning. Multidisciplinary senior staff meetings were also held regularly.
- Initial assessments involving the use of standardised assessments.
- Leisure therapy was encouraged daily in the form of gardening, craft work or outings for patients and relatives.
- Relatives and carer support group meetings and teaching sessions.

Apart from rehabilitation following the normal movement concept, the above procedures were not carried out on the conventional rehabilitation wards. Therefore, this description gives an overview of the philosophies, policies and procedures that were used on the Nottingham Stroke Unit but which were not present on the conventional rehabilitation wards.

Pertinent factors

From observations of patients' progress in rehabilitation, the pertinent factors which could affect positive stroke rehabilitation outcome appeared to be:

- Having established philosophies, polices and procedures that were applied by all disciplines, twenty-four hours per day.
- Having blanket referral, which allowed therapy to commence the moment the patient was admitted to the stroke unit.
- Having interdisciplinary working and a ward-based multidisciplinary team, with all treatment being carried out on the ward. All disciplines integrated and incorporated their knowledge and experience of each others' domains, within their specific area of treatment. Members of the multidisciplinary were therefore readily accessible, which facilitated improved communication and interaction between disciplines and multidisciplinary treatment sessions.
- Nursing integration with the rehabilitation team. The change in nurses' roles from the role of caring (*doing*) for patients to that of enabling (*facilitating*) patients facilitated a different outlook on nursing care. Nurses were able to concentrate on rehabilitation and were more aware of the problems resulting from a stroke and the treatment of these problems.
- The availability of staff from disciplines, such as speech and language therapists, clinical psychologists and dieticians.

These pertinent factors were observed by the author from her own clinical experiences, and their positive influence is supported by her anecdotal evidence. They describe the main aspects of care on the stroke unit involved in the Juby *et al* (1996), Drummond *et al* (1996) and Lincoln *et al*

(1997) studies. The combination of these pertinent factors may be responsible for the differences in outcome found in these studies. However, it should be remembered that this has not been proven through the use of appropriate research methodologies as being responsible for producing these differences.

Conclusion

There is little evidence to show what actually influences the effectiveness of stroke units. Pertinent differences between one stroke unit and the conventional rehabilitation wards in the same hospital appeared to include having established philosophies, polices and procedures that were applied by all disciplines, twenty-four hours per day and having the multidisciplinary team ward-based. It is most likely that the effectiveness of stroke units is dependent on this overall package of care and the large number of individual components that make up this package. It would be difficult to isolate any one or group of these components to identify their effectiveness. However, further investigation is still needed to try to identify which are the most important components that facilitate this effectiveness.

The author would like to thank Julia Webster, Senior Occupational Therapist, Nottingham City Hospital, for her assistance in preparing this paper.

References

Bobath B (1976) *Adult Hemiplegia: Evaluation and Treatment.* Heinemann, London

Brunnstrom S (1970) *Movement Therapy in Hemiplegia.* Harper and Row, London

Carr JH, Shepherd RB (1987) *A Motor Relearning Programme for Stroke.* 2nd edn. Heinemann Physio, London

Dennis M, Langhorne P (1994) So stroke units save lives: where do we go from here? *Br Med J* **309:** 1273–7

Drummond AER, Miller N, Colquohoun M, Logan PC (1996) The effects of a stroke unit on activities of daily living. *Clin Rehabil* **10:** 12–22

Garraway WM, Akhtar AJ, Hockey L, Prescott RJ (1980a) Management of acute stroke in the elderly — follow-up of a controlled trial. *Br Med J* **281:** 827–9

Garraway WM, Akhtar AJ, Prescott RJ, Hockey L (1980b) Management of acute stroke in the elderly: preliminary results of a controlled trial. *Br Med J* **280:** 1040–3

Goff B (1969) Appropriate afferent stimulation. *Physiotherapy* **55:** 9–17

Indredavik B, Bakke F, Solberg R, Rokseth R, Haheim L, Holme I (1991) Benefit of a stroke unit: a randomised controlled trial. *Stroke* **22:** 1026–31

Indredavik B, Slordahl SA, Bakke F, Rokseth R, Haheim LL (1997) Stroke unit treatment: long term effects. *Stroke* **28:** 1861–6

Indredavik B, Bakke F, Slordahl SA, Rokseth R, Haheim LL (1998) Stroke unit treatment improves long-term quality of life: a randomised controlled trial. *Stroke* **29:** 895–9

Indredavik B, Bakke F, Slordahl SA, Rokseth R, Haheim LL (1999a) Treatment in a combined acute and rehabilitation stroke unit, which aspects are most important. *Stroke* **30:** 917–23

Indredavik B, Bakke F, Slordahl SA, Rokseth R, Haheim LL (1999b) Stroke unit treatment: ten-year follow-up. *Stroke* **30:** 1524–7

Johnstone M (1980) *Home Care for the Stroke Patient: Living in a Pattern.* Churchill Livingstone, Edinburgh

Juby LC, Lincoln NB, Berman P (1996) The effect of a stroke rehabilitation unit on functional and psychological outcome: a randomised controlled trial. *Cerebrovasc Dis* **6:** 106–10

Kalra L, Dale P, Crome P (1993) Improving stroke rehabilitation. *Stroke* **24:** 1462–7

Kalra L, Eade J (1995) Role of stroke rehabilitation units in managing severe disability after stroke. *Stroke* **26:** 2031–4

King's Fund Consensus Conference (1988) Treatment of stroke. *Br Med J* **297:** 128

Knott M, Voss D (1968) *Proprioceptive Neuromuscular Facilitation.* 2nd edn. Harper and Row, London

Langhorne P (1997). The stroke unit story. *Stroke Matters* **1**(2): 1

Langhorne P, Dennis M (1998). *Stroke Units: an Evidence-based Approach.* BMJ Books, London

Langhorne P, Williams BO, Gilchrist W, Howie K (1993). Do stroke units save lives? *Lancet* **342:** 395–8

Lincoln NB, Drummond AER, Berman P (1997). Perceptual impairment and its impact on rehabilitation outcome. *Disabil Rehabil* **19**(6): 231–4

Lincoln NB, Willis D, Philips SA, Juby LC, Berman P (1996) Comparison of rehabilitation practice on hospital wards for stroke patients. *Stroke* **27:** 18–2

Ronning OM, Guldvog B (1998a) Stroke unit versus general medical wards. I: Twelve and eighteen month survival, a randomised controlled trial. *Stroke* **29:** 58–62

Ronning OM, Guldvog B (1998b) Stroke unit versus general medical wards. II: Neurological deficits and activities of daily living, a quasi-randomised controlled trial. *Stroke* **29:** 586–90

Smith ME, Garraway WM, Smith DL, Akhtar AJ (1982) Therapy impact of functional outcome in a controlled trial of stroke rehabilitation. *Arch Phys Med Rehabil* **63**: 21–24

Stevens RS, Ambler NR, Warren MD (1984) A randomised controlled trial of a stroke rehabilitation ward. *Age Ageing* **13:** 65–75

Stroke Unit Trialist's Collaboration (1997) Collaborative systematic review of the randomised trials of organised in-patient (stroke unit) care after stroke. *Br Med J* **314:** 1151–9

CHAPTER 8

Post-stroke physiotherapy in context

George Dowswell, Therese Dowswell, John Lawler, John Green, John Young

A year after stroke, it is unclear whether the provision of an additional course of physiotherapy has a beneficial impact on persistent stroke-related problems. This qualitative study identifies the views of patients and care-givers and discusses factors that may limit the effectiveness of further physiotherapy.

After a disabling stroke, most patients will receive rehabilitation services including physiotherapy (Ashburn *et al*, 1993). However, many stroke-related problems persist in the longer term, and early gains may not be sustained (Kettle and Chamberlain, 1989).

The primary aim of physiotherapy is usually to improve mobility and functional ability. Nevertheless, there is some evidence that while physiotherapists concentrate on patients regaining or maintaining physical capabilities, they also aim for recovery in a more holistic sense (Lewinter and Mikkelsen, 1995). Poor long-term outcomes have been documented in terms of physical and psychological well-being and social adjustment, and a number of studies have shown that patients are frequently disappointed with the extent of their recovery (Anderson, 1993; Evans *et al*, 1994; Pound *et al*, 1999). Persisting problems in stroke patients also have long-term consequences for informal care-givers (Wade *et al*, 1986; Greveson, 1991). While these longer-term, stroke-related problems are now better understood, appropriate and effective service responses have not yet been defined (Pound *et al*, 1998; Dowswell *et al*, 1997). Persisting mobility problems are particularly common (Ashburn *et al*, 1993). Therefore, one potentially helpful service response could be a further contact with a physiotherapy service at about one year after stroke onset.

In a previous study investigating the effects of physiotherapy one year after stroke, Wade *et al* (1992) used a range of quantitative outcome measures but demonstrated only a transient treatment effect. In this study, quantitative methods could not determine why the effect of rehabilitation was limited. Therefore, in the design of a second randomised controlled trial to evaluate late provision of physiotherapy to stroke patients with persisting mobility disability, a complementary qualitative study was incorporated and is reported in this paper.

The objectives of the qualitative study were twofold. First, the study sought to explore whether patients and care-givers perceive outcomes from a late physiotherapy intervention which have not been measured by standardised instruments. It is possible that there are positive effects of services that have not been recognised in quantitative studies. Second, the study sought to examine the context in which late physiotherapy services are delivered. This exploration would help uncover those patient and service factors that might limit or enhance the effect of a service intervention.

It was envisaged that the qualitative study would provide information that could be used to improve the quality of services to stroke patients. First, a recognition of those outcomes valued by patients and care-givers would enable service providers to design services explicitly to meet these ends and to incorporate these outcomes in evaluation instruments. Second, a recognition of those factors that constrain or enhance the impact of stroke services would enable service providers to target services more effectively so that only those patients in circumstances most likely to gain from late physiotherapy services receive them.

Background to the qualitative study

There has been a number of studies of patients' and care-givers' perspectives on the effects of stroke and the recovery process, along with their views about services after stroke. These studies of patients' and care-givers' perceptions of the early recovery period have shown that there are generally high levels of satisfaction with rehabilitation services (Intercollegiate Working Party for Stroke, 1998). Pound *et al* (1994) have described aspects of physiotherapy interventions appreciated by patients. For example, therapists were appreciated as a source of information, advice and support, as well as for bringing about specific functional improvements. It was also noted that patients perceived physiotherapy in terms of 'more being better' — ie. they believed that the more physiotherapy they received, the greater their functional improvement and overall recovery. This finding has also emerged elsewhere, although there has been little quantitative research to support this belief (Lewinter and Mikkelsen, 1995; Intercollegiate Working Party for Stroke, 1998). There is evidence that withdrawal of physiotherapy services is perceived as a loss for many patients, expressed as feelings of abandonment (Dowswell *et al*, 1997).

Qualitative studies of the aftermath of stroke have also drawn attention to the complexity of stroke recovery, with patients and health professionals using a variety of means to assess recovery (Trigg *et al*, 1999). However, while service providers and researchers have commonly emphasised physical recovery, patients and care-givers may not see physical gains as ends in their own right but as means of achieving more highly valued social, domestic and leisure pursuits. While patients may be aware of impairment and disability, handicap is the main level at which patients judge outcome (Pound *et al*, 1998; Hafsteindottir and Grypdonck, 1997). Most previous work has related to early physiotherapy services and to the weeks and months after stroke. It is not clear whether those outcomes valued by patients and care-givers are the same in the longer term.

Theoretical background

Complex interactions between physical and other domains of stroke recovery have been noted in both quantitative and qualitative research. Thus, recovery is a multidimensional concept, and at the individual level it takes place in a variety of contexts. While services may target very specific aspects of the recovery process, the service will be delivered under a wide variety of circumstances, by a diverse group of individuals and to a group of individuals all of whom have had strokes but otherwise may have very little in common (Ballinger *et al*, 1999).

Qualitative studies have identified the process of stroke recovery as one of coming to terms with loss, not only of physical function but also of social roles and identity. In some respects, recovery from stroke reflects the bereavement process that follows other major life events involving loss. Glass and Maddox (1992), drawing on the work of Parkes (1971), have described stroke recovery as a process of psychosocial transition. Stroke leads to major changes in individuals, in their social networks and in their interactions with others. Changes occur within two broad spheres. First, changes occur in what has been described as an individual's 'life space'. This includes the whole social and physical context in which individuals operate: their home, work and leisure environment, other people and their own bodies. Second, changes occur in what is referred to as the 'assumptive' world: the cultural and personal context within which individuals view their social world. The assumptive world is built up from previous experience and underpins all our interactions with others, forming the basis for our beliefs, expectations, interpretations and decisions. The two concepts are related. Thus, a major change in life space occurring as a result of stroke may challenge previously held assumptions and beliefs and provide a new context for forming expectations and for making plans and judgments. Successful adjustment depends on the individual altering and aligning their assumptive world with their altered life space.

This theoretical work is useful in thinking about health services and patients' and care-givers' views of services. Rehabilitation services seek to promote optimal physical recovery, along with successful adjustment to stroke. Thus, interventions need to target both problems associated with new life space (and this will include changes in the patient's physical condition) and problems in the patient's assumptive world (including unrealistic expectations of the recovery process). The concept of life space is also helpful in thinking about the potential and perceived contribution of services. Services are delivered within the context of patients' and care-givers' lives, which are constantly changing over time and which will differ in the immediate aftermath of stroke and in the longer term.

The key questions addressed by the qualitative study closely related to these issues. First, patients and care-givers were asked to discuss the effect of stroke and the process of recovery. They were asked to describe the experience of having a stroke and any changes they perceived in their lives since then. Second, they were asked to evaluate the contribution of a late physiotherapy intervention within the wider context of changes in their lives. They were asked about their expectations of services, their experience and to describe any positive and negative outcomes of the intervention.

Methods

This qualitative study was carried out as an adjunct to a randomised controlled trial examining the effects of a physiotherapy intervention one year after stroke. After approval of the trial by the local ethics committee, 170 patients were recruited from existing hospital and community rehabilitation service registers. Half were randomised to receive the physiotherapy intervention over a three-month period (treatment group). The others received no intervention (control group). Both groups were followed up every three months for nine months. In the randomised controlled trial, the primary outcome measure was the Rivermead Mobility Index (Collen *et al*, 1991). Other standardised instruments, including the Barthel Index (Mahoney and Barthel, 1965), the Frenchay Activities Index (Holbrook and Skilbeck, 1983) and the Hospital Anxiety and Depression Scale (Zigmond and Snaith, 1983), were also used.

Table 8.1: Patients participating in qualitative study (from physiotherapy records)

Sex	Male	15
	Female	5
Median age in years (range)		71 (54–81)
Stroke type	Left	6
	Right	12
	Other	2
Communication problems		2
Barthel – median (IQR, range)		18 (16–19; 10–20)
Months from stroke to interview – median (range)		25 (23–43)
Number of treatments – median (IQR, range)		5 (3–7; 1–17)

IQR = interquartile range

The physiotherapy intervention was delivered by a community physiotherapy service at the same time as their normal caseload. A problem-solving approach and a minimum of three contacts with each patient (Green *et al*, 1999) were agreed on by the physiotherapists.

At the end of physiotherapy treatment and follow-up, a purposeful sample of patients was drawn from the treatment group for the qualitative study. Patients were stratified according to initial mobility impairment (Rivermead Mobility Index 0–6; 7–11; 12–15) and geographical location. A sample reflecting the characteristics of the study population consisted of twenty patients with a range of stroke severity who had received physiotherapy from one of the four participating community rehabilitation centres. (Two of the original sample of patients declined to participate in the qualitative study. Two patients with similar characteristics were therefore selected to replace them.) If a principal care-giver resided with the patient, the care-giver was asked to participate in the study. All care-givers accepted this invitation. Written consent was obtained from all patients and care-givers.

Semi-structured interviews were carried out with patients and their care-givers (spouses and other relatives) by two interviewers between April 1998 and February 1999. Interviews with patients and care-givers took place separately but simultaneously. This allowed participants to speak without constraint or contradiction (Brannen and Collard, 1982). Interviews were carried out six to eight months after the physiotherapy intervention, approximately twenty-five months after the initial strokes. The interview schedule covered several main topic areas. It began with introductory questions about the patient's stroke and its effects and then moved on to services received. Questions were asked about any physiotherapy received in the last six to twelve months. Specific details of the physiotherapy were sought, followed by an evaluation of the physiotherapy. The interviews lasted between thirty and sixty minutes and were transcribed in full. Analysis was carried out using a qualitative data analysis package (NUD*IST). Each transcript was read several times by three members of the research team. A coding framework of broad response categories was developed to classify data, and constant comparison was used to refine classifications. Discussions within the research team led iteratively to the re-examination of the data in the light of emerging theoretical frameworks (Strauss and Corbin, 1990).

In addition, physiotherapy records were made available to the qualitative research team. These records provided demographic

Table 8.2: Physiotherapy contacts according to patients, care-givers and physiotherapy records

	Number of treatment sessions according to:			
Patient ID	Patient	Care-giver	Physiotherapy records	Total treatment time (h/min)
1	2	3	3	1h20
2	1	0	1	0h35
3	'weeks'	8+	10	6h50
4	8	0	7	5h35
5	8	14	17	15h15
6	3	n/a	5	2h20
7	2	2	2	0h50
8	0	n/a	7	4h00
9	1	missing	5	3h10
10	2	n/a	3	2h00
11	6	n/a	8	6h10
12	d/k	n/a	7	3h50
13	6	missing	3	1h35
14	6	n/a	5	2h30
15	0	n/a	4	2h00
16	0	n/a	2	1h30
17	8	missing	8	5h25
18	6	0	9	8h25
19	0	n/a	0	0h00
20	6	n/a	3	1h20

missing = no data available
d/k = 'don't know'

information about patients and details of the number and duration of the physiotherapy sessions that patients received. In the results section, verbatim accounts are used to illustrate the response categories.

Results

Twenty patients and ten care-givers were interviewed at home. Patient characteristics are set out in *Table 8.1*. One patient was found to have received no physiotherapy owing to administrative error. The remaining nineteen patients all received a home assessment visit from a community physiotherapist. After this, one patient refused further physiotherapy. Ten continued to receive physiotherapy at home and eight were treated as outpatients at a rehabilitation centre. According to physiotherapy records, the number of physiotherapy sessions varied considerably: median 5, minimum 0, maximum 17. The total amount of physiotherapy contact was similarly varied: mean 3 hours 44 minutes, minimum 0, maximum 15 hours and 15 minutes. There were also differences between patients' reports of the number of sessions they had received and physiotherapy service records (*Table 8.2*). Of the patients and care-givers who specified the number of treatment sessions received, twelve reported the same (plus or minus one) number of sessions as the physiotherapists, eleven reported fewer and two reported more than the records. There was no significant difference between the number of sessions or the total length of time of interventions in this sub-sample compared with the whole of the treatment group.

In the interviews, patients and care-givers described their lives before and after their stroke, experiences of the physiotherapy intervention, and their perceptions of its value. The three themes (lives, service context and evaluation) were interrelated and are set out in the three sections below.

The effects of stroke and coexisting illness

Patients and care-givers described in detail the circumstances in which stroke occurred and the immediate and enduring effects. As part of these accounts, patients described other health changes occurring since their stroke (which may or may not have been related to the stroke). Patients and care-givers described the diverse nature of the experience of having a stroke. Some patients lost consciousness and were hospitalised immediately, while others felt unwell but did not seek medical attention for some days or were not referred for hospital care. Strokes occurred in the context of lives that were very different, and the immediate experience of the stroke was mediated by individual characteristics (eg. stroke severity and age) and circumstances (activities, social networks and home environment).

> *It were quarter to one in the morning. I went to the club celebrating my birthday. I used to drink a lot. I'd had thirty bottles of Budweiser and fifteen double vodkas, because all of my mates had been buying them, and I was dancing... dancing with my mate's wife, because my wife doesn't drink, and I just fell along the table and all the drinks went. I thought I was drunk. I thought, 'I've never been this drunk before'... I was like trying to stand up but I couldn't... this woman came across and said, 'Don't be banging him about it looks like he's had a stroke.' So they phoned an ambulance and took me to hospital.*
>
> Male patient, age 54, ID11

> *When it first started, you know, I was going across the road, I always went for my own paper in the morning, and went across the road, and I was sludging [sic] this left foot. And that was it.*
>
> Male patient, age 81, ID3

While some of the longer-term consequences of the stroke were common to most of the sample, the ways that these affected aspects of patients' and care-givers' lives were mediated by individual circumstances. Problems with limb movement, balance, speech and memory were mentioned by several. Patients with fairly minor physical impairment described serious psychological effects of stroke and their lack of confidence in terms of resuming pre-stroke roles and activities. Patients and care-givers also referred to good and bad days, as though the effect of stroke varied on a daily basis as well as over longer periods. Stroke affected bodies and minds, roles and relationships.

It's hard to say, I've lost all my confidence, and I think I became a hypochondriac sort of thing. It certainly took a bit of the wind out of my sails. It made you realise, you know, you're over fifty and you're getting older.

Male patient, age 55, ID12

I can't bend down, it's very awkward picking things up. I don't know why, but sometimes the wife has to put my stockings on. I can't put them on properly. I can do — I put them on myself this morning because she went out for pension.

Male patient, age 72, ID13

With the speech and her memory, and all her right side. She still hasn't got full use of her right side. She's not right clever at walking yet. Everything. She's completely changed from what she used to be. She doesn't want to do anything. I've got to force her, more or less, to do things. She used to do a lot of knitting, gardening, stuff like that. I'm doing it, more or less all now, the housework and everything. That's how it's affected her.

Male care-giver, ID7c

Several patients and care-givers described coexisting illness. This was sometimes a continuation from pre-stroke life, a consequence or 'side-effect' of stroke, or it was simply put down to old age. Seven patients said that they had experienced a fall in the last year, and seven described other health problems that they thought had hindered their stroke recovery. Concurrent health problems included cancer, diabetes, arthritis and back pain, angina, weight gain, asthma and 'nerves'. Thus, the physiotherapy intervention was offered to patients with different experiences of stroke at different stages in the recovery process, with varied health states and with different perspectives on which physical impairments created handicap in their lives.

The physiotherapy intervention

In addition to the wide variation in health states, late physiotherapy was offered to patients who had had varied experiences of health services in the aftermath of stroke. Twelve patients described receiving physiotherapy soon after their strokes, and all had received interventions by other healthcare professionals (in community and hospital settings), including speech and occupational therapists and family doctors, along with social care workers. This experience of early interventions may have influenced patients' and care-givers' expectations and views of any later intervention (as experience and previously acquired knowledge form the basis for interpretation and views). Not all interventions had been appreciated, although most patients and care-givers held positive views about early service interventions. Regarding late physiotherapy, three of the twenty patients could not remember receiving any recent intervention at all, and one patient said that it had been offered but had been refused.

For the rest, the intervention varied in terms of content, provider, location and duration (*Tables 8.2* and *8.3*). Some patients did not distinguish between the physiotherapy intervention and the follow-up visits by a researcher to evaluate the effects of the intervention. Patients and care-givers describe sessions lasting between five and forty-five minutes and spread over between two and eight sessions. Sessions were delivered at home or at community healthcare venues by a range of staff.

I went once a week. It were a bit hit and miss. I would go three or four times, and then they'd suspend it. I just went for half an hour once a week. I think I would have been better with two periods a week, but I never asked for it. You could see they were busy. She [the therapist] would be talking to other people, it weren't her fault.

Male patient, age 76, ID4

Yes, that woman came… She came, the first time she came she said, 'I can't stop because I've got to go see, I've arranged to see somebody else at a certain time,' and she went off. She came twice — I think she came twice. And the second time, she were going on her holidays.

Female patient, age 62, ID7

The actual content of the intervention also varied. Some patients described walking indoors or outdoors; others described particular exercises or using special equipment; and some could not remember, or said they had just talked. One patient described being given written information by the physiotherapist and another a back massage.

The effects of the intervention in the context of lives

In view of the very varied accounts about the intervention, patients and care-givers perceived a variety of effects. Four of the patients claimed that the intervention had had no beneficial effect. Eleven said that the intervention had had some positive effect, but what patients valued about the intervention varied. Four described changes in mobility or movement, and this opened up the possibility of fulfiling roles or undertaking tasks that had been otherwise inaccessible, such as visiting shops or relatives. In addition, however, there was a range of other beneficial effects, such as increasing confidence, enjoying a trip out and feeling that someone was interested.

The perceived value of the intervention seemed to depend not only on the success of the intervention in bringing about improvements in physical abilities, but also on increases in their ability to pursue valued activities. However, the intervention was received in the context of patients' and care-givers' more general hopes and expectations of recovery. None of the patients evaluated the intervention outside this context. When asked about the effects of the intervention, patients did not speak of changes in movement alone but of the impact of the intervention within their lives as a whole. This led to a contradiction: while patients and care-givers could point to some benefits in terms of physical capacity, the overall value of the intervention was nevertheless limited. The intervention was short and focused on discrete outcomes. From the patients' perspectives, recovery was a long-term holistic process. Patients and care-givers recognised that returning to

Table 8.3: Nature of physiotherapy intervention

Nineteen patients had a total of 109 sessions of physiotherapy with 231 separate elements noted in physiotherapists' records

	Number	%
Gait re-education	86	37
Exercise therapy	35	15
Balance re-education	26	11
Functional exercises	22	10
Patient assessment	20	9
Neurological mobilisation	16	7
Electrotherapy for other conditions	12	5
Upper limb treatment	7	3
Counselling/advice	4	2
Other*	3	1
Total	**231**	

*Other included supply of stick, review and posture re-education

pre-stroke roles and relationships was an ambitious hope, and the impact of therapy on the process as a whole was limited. Two of the care-givers and several patients included the expression 'working miracles' in their accounts. A recognition of the limitations of the service in terms of achieving major changes in the patient's condition, physical or otherwise, was implicit in most accounts. This does not mean that small changes were not valued but that their value depended on the wider context.

But it got my leg going. When you are like this, you appreciate a hundred yards. You forget about owt [anything] else, as long as you can walk to the gate... I haven't got worse, that's what I mean... I'd have liked to have got my arms going, I can't even fasten my laces... I enjoyed it. Going for a ride [in the ambulance] and that. And I'd do anything they asked me to do — what I could do, you know. But you can't do impossibilities, can you?... I didn't want miracles, because I know they wouldn't happen. I expected what they had on the menu, you know.

Male patient, age 70, ID1

Interviewer (GD): *Was the physiotherapy you had at [the centre], was it of any value?*
Interviewee (Male patient, age 79, ID18): *Well, I think it was, but as I said, it would be limited value because we're working on a duff steer [a hopeless case], so to speak... Let's face it, don't lose sight of the fact I'm seventy nine... I'd just put the point that I think therapy is very, very useful, given the right conditions and the right situation, but it's a little bit awkward — it doesn't seem very fair asking a therapist to make a dead man walk, for example.*

It gave me the confidence to do things. To go for a walk, to go to the Co-op.

Female patient, age 60, ID20

Well, likes of me, I think they have done what they can for me. This is as far as they can take me... I think I am going to be more or less like this, and that is it. But I think they have brought me quite far. You know what I can do and cannot do, on a nice day.

Male patient, age 55, ID12

None of the patients had resumed what they perceived as their normal lives almost two years or more after the stroke. There had been some changes in patients' physical condition during the post-stroke period, but no-one made what they perceived to be a full recovery. Changes in life space were, for all of this sample, major, largely negative, and enduring.

Discussion

These twenty patients described a wide variation in their pre-stroke lives, in their experiences of stroke, in the immediate aftermath of stroke, and in the months and years after the stroke. These varied lives were used as a context to evaluate service interventions. Late rehabilitation services were valued by patients on a number of counts. Only four patients pointed to improvements in discrete movements as a valued outcome. The most valued outcomes related to wider goals and the ability to pursue valued activities.

The study had a number of limitations. The sample was not large (twenty patients and ten care-givers) and was drawn from a particular geographical area. On the other hand, the sample was diverse, including patients with varied health states, of different ages and from a variety of social backgrounds. The interviews were carried out more than twenty months after stroke and at least six months since treatment, which probably had some impact on recall. Some of the patients had memory and speech difficulties, and this may have affected responses. Nevertheless, patients and care-givers provided rich accounts of their experience of stroke and the impact of interventions which have implications for stroke research, stroke services and for the way that services are evaluated.

The study illustrated the complexity of stroke recovery as a social transition. It highlighted the many variables that affect recovery and perceptions about services. It also showed that if service interventions attempt to address individual needs, then they are likely to be extremely varied. Variability in service provision is often appropriate, as providers will use their professional judgment to tailor services to meet what they perceive as the needs of particular patients. Professional judgment may include an assessment of the context in which services will be received. However, a difficulty with providing a context-specific intervention is that service evaluation then becomes difficult.

In health services research, controlling the content of an experimental intervention is a tall order. The intervention described in this study was not uniform. Patients received very different amounts of service interventions, and their content varied. In randomised controlled trials, the division into control and intervention groups is carried out to take account of chance variation in the target population. However, variation in the intervention is often not acknowledged. Thus, analysis is often a simple comparison between groups carried out on an 'intention to treat' basis. Unless researchers explicitly acknowledge that there is variation in process, then linking services with outcome is problematic and answering questions, such as what type of intervention is beneficial and under what circumstances, remains difficult.

This study and others have shown that the effects of intervention, while beneficial, may not be large or the intended ones. Patients varied before the intervention occurred, the interventions were relatively minor and short-lived, and what individuals perceived as valuable also varied. Given this diversity, it is not surprising that researchers find it difficult to detect meaningful treatment effects in randomised trials. The collection of qualitative data on outcomes may be a worthwhile addition in a quantitative trial.

Stroke adjustment has much in common with the grieving process, but differs from it in that the loss is variable, changes to life space are diverse, and losses may not be permanent. This has implications for patients' assumptions and beliefs. Acceptance of changes in life space are tempered and possibly obstructed by enduring but potentially irrational hopes. While patients' expectations of the intervention were limited and probably self-fulfilling, their hopes relating to taking up previous roles and activities were more ambitious.

In short, the problems arising from stroke were serious, long-standing and varied, while the interventions were of short duration and dealt with only limited aspects of service-defined problems. Patients' aims were not mobility or gait speed — they were at the level of handicap. Interventions have to be intensively targeted at that level to achieve positive changes in patients' lives. The study also showed that there were continuing problems with adjustment to stroke. While patients and care-givers had realistic expectations about services and realised that physiotherapy was unlikely to achieve miracles, they nevertheless felt disappointed with their recovery. The experience of stroke had not led to major changes in patients' assumptive worlds. These are issues that must be addressed in the goal-setting process with patients.

Conclusions

To ensure that sustained improvements result from physiotherapy services a year after stroke, attention must be paid to a number of factors highlighted by this qualitative study. First, at the simplest level, there is a case for patients who regard themselves as 'duff steers' or as being unable to participate fully because of old age or specific comorbidity being excluded from research studies examining service effectiveness. Stroke services can thus be targeted at those individuals who are able to benefit from them.

Second, patients must perceive the intervention as worthwhile; that is, they must receive what they regard as a substantial amount of focused, individual attention for a considerable period of time. Patients' expectations of what the intervention will involve and its potential outcomes must be explored at an early stage. Then steps must be taken to address doubts or identify and challenge negative views to ensure full participation on a positive basis. If patients cannot be convinced that physiotherapy is substantial and potentially beneficial, it seems unlikely that they can benefit.

Third, patients have to be convinced that they have a positive part to play in partnership with physiotherapists.

The majority of patients could identify some positive feature of their involvement in this research project. The extent to which they gained continuing benefit from it appeared to be dependent on patients' perceptions of whether there was real scope for improvement in their condition, and their confidence in the capacity of the service intervention to achieve it.

The authors would like to thank the Stroke Association for funding the study and the patients, care-givers and physiotherapist without whom the study would not have been possible.

References

Anderson R (1993) *The Aftermath of Stroke: the Experience of Patients and Their Families.* Cambridge University Press, Cambridge

Ashburn A, Partridge C, De Souza L (1993) Physiotherapy in the rehabilitation of stroke: a review. *Clin Rehabil* **7**: 337–45

Ballinger C, Ashburn A, Low J, Roderick P (1999) Unpacking the black-box of therapy — a pilot study to describe occupational and physiotherapy interventions for people with stroke. *Clin Rehabil* **13**: 301–9

Brannen J, Collard T (1982) *Marriage in Trouble: the Process of Seeking Help.* Tavistock Institute, London

Collen FM, Wade DT, Robb GF, Bradshaw CM (1991) The Rivermead Mobility Index: a further development of the Rivermead Motor Assessment. *Int Disabil Stud* **13**: 50–4

Dowswell G, Lawler J, Young J, Forster A, Hearn J (1997) A qualitative study of specialist nurse support for stroke patients and care-givers at home. *Clin Rehabil* **11**: 293–301

Evans RL, Connis RT, Bishop DS, Hendrick RD, Haselkorn JK (1994) Stroke: a family dilemma. *Disabil Rehabil* **16**(3): 110–18

Glass TA, Maddox GL (1992) The quality and quantity of social support: stroke recovery as psycho-social transition. *Soc Sci Med* **34**(11): 1349–61

Green JR, Forster A, Young J (1999) A survey of community physiotherapy provision after 1 year post-stroke. *Br J Ther Rehabil* **6**: 216–21

Greveson G (1991) Improving long-term outcome after stroke — the views of patients and care-givers. *Health Trends* **23**(4): 161–2

Hafsteindottir TB, Grypdonck M (1997) Being a stroke patient: a review of the literature. *J Adv Nurs* **26**: 580–8

Holbrook ME, Skilbeck CE (1983) An activities index for use with stroke patients. *Age Ageing* **12**: 166–70

Intercollegiate Working Party for Stroke (1998) *Stroke Rehabilitation. Patient and Care-giver Views.* College of Health and Royal College of Physicians, London

Kettle M, Chamberlain MA (1989) The stroke patient in an urban environment. *Clin Rehabil* **3**: 131–8

Lewinter M, Mikkelsen S (1995) Therapists and the rehabilitation process after stroke. *Disabil Rehabil* **17**(5): 211–16

Mahoney FI, Barthel DW (1965) Functional evaluation: the Barthel Index. *Md State Med J* **14**: 61–5

Parkes CM (1971) Psycho-social transitions: a field of study. *Soc Sci Med* **5**: 101–15

Pound P, Bury M, Gompertz P, Ebrahim S (1994) Views of the survivors of stroke on benefits of physiotherapy. *Qual Health Care* **3**: 69–74

Pound P, Gompertz P, Ebrahim S (1998) A patient-centred study of the consequences of stroke. *Clin Rehabil* **12**: 338–47

Pound P, Tilling K, Rudd AG, Wolfe CDA (1999) Does patient satisfaction reflect differences in care received after stroke? *Stroke* **30**: 49–55

Strauss A, Corbin J (1990) *Basics of Qualitative Research: Grounded Theory, Procedures and Techniques*. Sage, London

Trigg R, Wood VA, Langton Hewer R (1999) Social reintegration after stroke: the first stages in the development of the Subjective Index of Physical and Social Outcome (SIPSO). *Clin Rehabil* **13**: 341–53

Wade DT, Leigh Smith J, Langton Hewer R (1986) Effects of living with and looking after survivors of stroke. *Br Med J* **293**: 418–20

Wade DT, Collen FM, Robb GF, Warlow CP (1992) Physiotherapy intervention late after stroke and mobility. *Br Med J* **304**: 609–13

Zigmond AS, Snaith RP (1983) The Hospital Anxiety and Depression Scale. *Acta Psychiatr Scand* **67**: 361–70

CHAPTER 9

Post-stroke depression

Angela Gall

Depression following stroke is common. Although it is highlighted as an issue in stroke guidelines, guidance on diagnosis or management is not given. This chapter presents the original research from a literature review of Medline and the Cochrane Database on stroke and depression, and discusses some of the clinical implications of the findings.

Mood disturbance following stroke can take several forms. This chapter will mainly discuss depression — its incidence, clinical features, associations and therapeutic options. The chapter also briefly considers emotional lability, which is also relatively common and can be mistaken for depression. Adjustment reactions, abnormal illness behaviour, adoption of the 'sick role' or institutionalisation and anxiety disorder can also occur after stroke, but these are not specifically dealt with here.

Clinical significance

Post-stroke depression (PSD) can present as an obstacle to rehabilitation. It has an independent negative effect on longer-term recovery of physical function (Berg *et al*, 2003; Gainotti *et al*, 2001; Pohjasvaara *et al*, 2001), cognition (Morris *et al*, 1992) and social function (Clark and Smith, 1998). Patients who are depressed tend to stay in hospital longer. There is also evidence of a significant relationship between depressive symptoms and stroke mortality (Everson *et al*, 1998; House *et al*, 2001), even after adjustments for age, sex, race and risk factors (Williams *et al*, 2004). Although in 60% of patients the depression will resolve at twelve months irrespective of treatment, those in whom it has not will have a high risk of chronic depression (Astrom *et al*, 1993). One study has examined the incidence of suicide following stroke and reported a significantly increased risk, especially in females and in those less than sixty years-old (Stenager *et al*, 1998; Cassidy *et al*, 2004). It might be argued that formal assessment of suicide risk in any patient with depressive symptoms should be included in all stroke-management protocols.

Table 9.1: Suggested risk factors for post-stroke depression

No proven association	Increased risk	Odds ratio
Age of patient	Female patients	n/a
Volume of the lesion	Past history of depressive illness	2.3–2.9
Side of the stroke	Increased impairment	n/a
Pathological type of stroke	Increased disability	1.8–2.9
Aetiology of stroke	Increased handicap	n/a
Location of lesion	Patients with dysphasia	n/a
	Patients living alone	n/a
	Patients with little social contact outside the home	n/a
	Cerebral atrophy on scan increases risk of depression at 3 years	n/a

n/a = data not available

Incidence

Several studies have examined the incidence of depression following stroke with different results. Most studies excluded patients with dysphasia and patients with moderate or severe cognitive impairments, although one group of researchers has developed a questionnaire for carers as a proxy for patients with dysphasia (Sutcliffe and Lincoln, 1998). Incidence rates between 5.6% and 55% have been reported (Morris *et al*, 1992; Astrom *et al*, 1993; Burvill *et al*, 1995; Pohjasvaara, 1998; Herrmann *et al*, 1998; Kotila *et al*, 1998; Verdello *et al*, 2004; Berg *et al*, 2001, 2003). Reasons for this wide variation may lie in differences in the diagnostic tools used; in the timing of the assessment following stroke; and in patient selection. The incidence of depression is reported higher in hospital (22–55%) than in community studies (11–25%).

Clinical associations

Several studies have examined risk factors for the development of depression following stroke (*Table 9.1*). Groups of patients at higher risk have been identified, and perhaps increased awareness will allow earlier diagnosis and treatment.

Aetiology

The aetiology of depressive illness in general is the subject of much research; it is evident that genetics, personality traits and the environment all contribute. Aben *et al* (2002) found that neuroticism was an important predictor of PSD. The monoamine neurotransmitters noradrenaline, serotonin and dopamine and their receptors have been widely studied and indirect evidence from the response of pharmacological agents acting on these pathways suggest a role in the aetiology of depressive illness (Gelder *et al*, 1996).

The specific aetiology of PSD has also been studied. It has been postulated that the psychological reaction to disability and social handicap has a role. Depression occurs more than twice as often following stroke than in age- and sex-matched controls (Wade *et al*, 1987; Burvill *et al*, 1995) and is more common following stroke than in other populations matched for physical disability. Folstein *et al* (1977) found that stroke patients were

Table 9.2: Symptoms of depressive order

Low mood and feeling of misery	
Loss of interest and pleasure from activities	
Pessimistic thinking	Past
	Present
	Future: may lead to hopelessness and suicidal ideation
Biological features	Energy loss
	Sleep disturbance
	Diurnal variation of mood
	Anorexia and weight loss
	Loss of libido
Psychotic features	Delusions: guilt, worthlessness, nihilism
	Hallucinations: auditory, persecutory

significantly more depressed than orthopaedic patients with equal levels of disability. Therefore, it seems unlikely that adjustment issues are the only cause, but it does not exclude the possibility that there may be specific adjustment issues in stroke.

There is no consistent evidence of any relationship to lesion location. Abnormalities in serotonin pathways have been suggested as causal factors. Lower levels of the serotonin metabolite 5-hydroxy indoleacetic acid (5HIAA) have been found in the cerebrospinal fluid of depressed compared with non-depressed stroke patients (Bryer *et al*, 1992). Patients following stroke have reduced serotoninergic responsiveness (prolactin response to d-fenluramine) when compared with controls (Ramasubbu *et al*, 1998; Morris *et al*, 2003). More work is required to improve our understanding of PSD; further understanding of the biochemical abnormalities may allow targeted pharmacological therapies to be developed.

Clinical assessment

The common symptoms and signs of depressive disorder in general are shown in *Tables 9.2* and *9.3* (Gelder *et al*, 1996). The difficulty in the diagnosis of depression following stroke will be apparent from these tables. Facial weakness can look similar to an unhappy expression; movement and function may be reduced; impairments of speech and language cause difficulty in assessing thoughts; cognitive impairments may be a direct consequence of the stroke lesion, particularly the apathy that can occur following frontal lesions. The atypical ward environment can confound the assessment: eating habits are changed; sleep disturbance is common; and patients may be adjusting to their new abilities — or merely bored. This difficulty in clinical diagnosis has led some to explore the use of formal assessment tools to assist in the diagnosis of depression following stroke.

Assessment tools

The 'gold standard' in the diagnosis of general depression is the Present State Examination (Helzer, 1983). This requires training to administer and is time-consuming. Other scales have been developed. These tools are not diagnostic; most are designed to screen for high-risk patients who warrant further assessment. Some have been developed for use in physically ill patients, but few have been validated in stroke. Assessment tools in stroke must allow for the physical symptoms that may exist as a result of the stroke itself, and must also allow for patients who may have language or cognitive impairments limiting the ability to complete the questionnaire. *Table 9.4* shows some of the tools currently used and quotes sensitivity, specificity, positive predictive value and misclassification rate for their use following stroke, where available.

There is no ideal assessment tool. The Hospital Anxiety and Depression Scale (HADS), General Depression Scale 15 and General Health Questionnaire are probably most commonly used. The General Depression Scale 15 has been recommended by the Royal College of Physicians as a useful screening tool for depression in elderly patients. Although it has been used in medical rehabilitation settings, there are, as yet, no data available on its use in stroke. Perhaps the HADS is the preferred tool, as it is short and relatively easy to complete: this is an important consideration if it is to be used as a screening tool, although the thresholds may be better set at 6–7 in the stroke population. As there is no gold standard for diagnosis, treatment may have to be considered on the basis of these 'screening tools'. Further studies are required to validate threshold HADS scores in relation to specific treatments. The use of care pathways may aid identification and management (Turner-Stoke and Hassan, 2002).

Table 9.3: Mental state examination

Appearance/behaviour	Looks unhappy, may be tearful, avoids eye contact
	May appear neglected
	Psychomotor retardation, slumped posture
	Agitation, irritability, sleep disturbance or reaction to perceptual disturbance may be observed
Speech	Slow, soft, lacks expression
Mood	Low mood, flat effect with lack of reactivity
Thoughts	Depressive themes
	May include suicidal ideation or delusions
Cognition	Impairments on formal testing, particularly concentration

Table 9.4: Tools used for assessment post-stroke

Assessment tool	References	Notes	Sens	Spec	PPV	MR
Hospital Anxiety and Depression Scale (HADS)	Zigmond and Snaith (1983), Abiodun (1994), Burvill et al (1995), Spinhoven et al (1997), O'Rourke et al (1998)	Validated in primary care and medical patients. Weighted to psychological symptoms. Gives probability of disorder				
		Cut off 3–4	94%	32%	25%	56%
		Cut off 4–5	83%	44%	26%	48%
		Cut off 6–7	83%	8%		
General Health Questionnaire (28) (GHQ)	Burvill et al (1995), Bridges and Goldberg (1986)	Screening tool for primary care and medical patients. Takes <10 minutes. Expressed as judgment of psychiatrist as case or non-case. Cut off 5–6	78%	81%	50%	20%
General Health Questionnaire (30)	O'Rourke et al (1998)	Cut off 8–9	80%	76%		
Montgomery Asberg Depression Rating Scale	Montgomery and Asberg (1979)	10 themes, 4-point scale for each. Interviewer has definitions. Psychological symptoms rated				
Beck Depression Inventory (BDI)	Beck et al (1961)	21-item patient completion scale. 4–6 statements per item. Cut off 9–10	92%	75%		
Geriatric Depression Scale (GDS 30)	Yesavage et al (1982–3), Burvill et al (1995)	30-item scale, cut off 10–11. Simple to administer, no trained interview skills required	84%	66%	53%	28%
15-item Geriatric Depression Scale (GDS 15)	Lesher and Berryhill (1994)	15-item scale — shorter form of GDS 30, validated reliability compared with GDS 30. Not studied in stroke				
Visual analogue scales	Davies et al (1975)	Mark along 10cm line as marker of mood				
Stroke Aphasia Depression questionnaire	Sutcliffe and Lincoln (1998)	Carer completes as proxy for dysphasic patients. Correlates with HADS. 21 items validated a 10-item version. Detects mood, not syndrome or prediction of treatment response				

Sens = sensitivity; spec = specificity; PPV = positive predictive value; MR = misclassification rate

Treatment options

Conservative management

Evidence from several studies indicates that there is a tendency for PSD to improve spontaneously over time. At two to six weeks following stroke, 50% of patients in one study improved independently of treatment, although spontaneous recovery after seven weeks was infrequent (Andersen *et al*, 1994). Approximately 50% of patients in another study who were depressed at three weeks or six months were no longer depressed at one

Table 9.5: Side-effects and drug interactions of tricyclic antidepressants

Side-effects	Anticholinergic	Dry mouth, tachycardia, blurred vision, urinary retention, constipation, erectile dysfunction, cognitive impairment
	Alpha IR block	Drowsiness, postural hypertension, cognitive impairment
	Antihistamine	Drowsiness, weight gain
	Cardiotoxic	Conduction defects, arrhythmias
	Lowers seizure threshold	
	Risk in overdose	
Drug interactions	Increased risk arrhythmias with antiarrhythmic drugs	
	Anticholinergic/antihistamine effects increased by concomitant use	
	Hypotensive effect antihypertensives increased	

year (Wade *et al*, 1987); another study reported a slightly higher recovery rate of 60% at one year (Astrom *et al*, 1993). Despite evidence that spontaneous recovery occurs, conservative management may allow depression to hamper the rehabilitation process needlessly.

Rehabilitation process

The rehabilitation process itself may also bring about improvement by maximising independence, increasing social stimulation, and relieving pain and other unpleasant symptoms (Wade, 1992). One study showed that a leisure rehabilitation programme had a beneficial effect on mood measured by the Nottingham Health Profile, although not when measured by the Wakefield Depression Inventory (Drummond and Walker, 1996).

Stroke family care worker

A randomised controlled trial (RCT) (Dennis *et al*, 1997) has examined the impact of a stroke family care worker on various outcomes following stroke. The worker had a social work

Table 9.6: Side-effects and drug interactions of selective serotonin-reuptake inhibitors

Side-effects	Common	Gastrointestinal	Nausea, anorexia, constipation, diarrhoea
		Central nervous system	Headache, dizziness, insomnia, restlessness
	Other	Sweating, anorgasmia, ejaculatory delay	
	5HT syndrome	Especially if use lithium/5HT$_1$ agonists	
Drug interactions		May inhibit hepatic metabolism tricyclics, antipsychotics and anticonvulsants	
		Effect of warfarin may be increased	

5HT = 5-hydroxytryptamine

background and was able to identify unmet needs; access health, social and voluntary services; and provide a counselling role. The treatment group expressed significantly greater satisfaction than the control group in certain aspects of their care. However, there were no differences in physical or mood-related outcomes in patients or carers.

Cognitive behavioural therapy

Cognitive behavioural therapy is of proven benefit in depressive illness. Its effect in PSD has been studied using Beck Depression Inventory and HADS (Lincoln *et al*, 1997). Severe strokes were excluded. The Beck Depression Inventory suggested a significant benefit, although the HADS or activities of daily living (ADL) score did not. The study was not controlled. A randomised controlled study by Licoln *et al* (2003) did not show any benefit of CBT following stroke. Further controlled studies are required to identify which patients are able to engage in cognitive behavioural therapy and are most likely to benefit.

Drug treatments

The treatments for depression following stroke are similar to those for other depressive illnesses and the use of antidepressant drugs after stroke is common (Eriksson *et al*, 2004).

Tricyclic antidepressants

These inhibit the reuptake of noradrenaline and serotonin. They are inexpensive, well-studied and have no proven long-term toxicity. Side-effects are common and often limit therapeutic treatment (*Table 9.5*). A double-blind placebo-controlled RCT (Lipsey *et al*, 1984) compared nortriptyline to placebo in thirty-four patients with PSD measured by the Hamilton Depression Scale (HDS), Zung Depression Score (ZDS) and Present State Examination. There was a significant beneficial effect of treatment by three weeks, which persisted at six weeks. Drop-out rates were comparable.

A double-blind randomised treatment trial in preventing PSD (Narushima *et al*, 2002) reported that both nortriptyline and fluoxetine appeared to be effacious, although nortriptyline produced an increased vulnerability to depression for more than six months after discontinuation.

Selective serotonin-reuptake inhibitors (SSRIs)

Selective serotonin-reuptake inhibitors (SSRIs) are attractive because a therapeutic level is soon reached. As they are a relatively recent development, their long-term effects are unknown. They have a less serious side-effect profile but gastrointestinal side-effects can be troublesome and they have more potential drug interactions (*Table 9.6*). Freuhwald *et al* (2003) reported the advantage of fluoxetine at eighteen months' follow-up in reducing relapse rate, but not over placebo as a treatment within the first three months.

The efficacy and safety of citalopram has been tested in PSD using a double-blind placebo-controlled RCT (Andersen *et al*, 1994). Thirty-three patients were in each arm, with a diagnosis of depression using the HDS. Benefits were seen in the treatment group at three and six weeks, although their drop-out rate was greater as a result of side-effects. (Of those entering in the study two to six weeks following their stroke, half recovered within one month, independently of treatment. In those entering more than seven weeks after the stroke, recovery was infrequent in the placebo group.)

The tolerability and efficacy of sertaline in the treatment as well as the prevention of PSD has been reported in different studies (Rasmassen *et al*, 2003; Zifko *et al*, 2002). The effect of fluoxetine in the prevention of PSD has been shown (Narushima *et al*, 2002).

Atypical antidepressants

Reding *et al* (1986) studied the effect of trazodone *vs* placebo in a twenty-seven-patient RCT, involving patients who were seen an average of forty-four days after they had had a stroke. There was no difference in drop-out rate between the groups. In patients with a clinical diagnosis of PSD or abnormal ZDSs, there was a tendency for Barthel Index scores to improve in the treatment group, although this did not reach statistical significance. There was no difference in side-effect rate.

The therapeutic effects of milnacipran, a serotonin and noradrenaline reuptake inhibitor, on PSD were studied by Kimura *et al* (2002) and the results suggested that it may be effective. Prophylactic mianserin had no beneficial effect on mood or function in a randomised, placebo-controlled study of 100 consecutive patients following stroke (Palomaki *et al*, 1999). Venlafaxine has been shown to be safe and tolerable in a small uncontrolled study by Dahmen *et al* (1999); ten of the twelve patients had a >50% reduction in HADS score following treatment. Evidence for a therapeutic effect must await a controlled study.

Stimulant drugs

Stimulants have also been studied in PSD. In a twenty-one-patient RCT, Grade *et al* (1998) showed that methylphenidate was beneficial in improving HDS, ZDS and the Functional Independence Measure. Methylphenidate has also been shown to be as effective as nortriptyline in improving depressive symptoms, with a significantly earlier effect: two to four days compared with twenty-seven days (Lazarus *et al*, 1994). An RCT found dextroamphetamine to be as effective as methylphenidate in improving mood (Masand *et al*, 1991).

Few data exist on optimal duration of therapy; this warrants further investigation. The three RCTs using antidepressant medication have outcomes at six weeks, although the optimal duration of therapy is likely to be longer if experience from depressive illness in general is relevant.

When considering pharmacological therapy, it is important to be aware of the possible effects on recovery and plasticity, although there are few data from human trials. A study comparing the effects of fluoxetine and maprotiline following stroke found a difference in recovery between the two groups, suggesting fluoxetine may facilitate or maprotiline may hinder recovery in post-stroke patients (Dam *et al*, 1996). Further studies suggest serotoninergic agents may have different effects on outcomes than noradrenergic agents, another area with potentially exciting new developments.

Electroconvulsive therapy

Electroconvulsive therapy can be indicated in severe depressive illness with biological or psychotic features. It is conceivable that stimulating seizure activity in subacutely injured brain may have different consequence from its use in the general depressive-illness population. Two retrospective studies have reported beneficial treatment effects in 86% and 95% of stroke patients. The safety and tolerability differ between the studies: one of fourteen adverse events occurred in the study by Murray *et al* (1986) and twelve of twenty suffered significant side-effects in Currier *et al*'s study in 1992 — seven relapsed on medical maintenance; five had medical complications (including hypertension, acute pulmonary oedema, multiple ventricular arrhythmias and severe interictal delirium — all in patients with pre-existing cardiovascular disease); and three developed confusion or amnesia. There are no prospective studies looking at the effect and safety of electroconvulsive therapy in PSD. The safety in PSD is therefore not established and an RCT looking at the therapeutic effect, as well as safety and tolerability, seems overdue.

Recent developments

Jorge *et al* (2004) did a randomised, parallel, double-blind study of active *vs* sham left prefrontal repetitive transcranial magnetic stimulation (rTMS) in patients with refractory PSD. After discontinuing antidepressant medication, patients were randomly assigned to receive ten sessions of active or sham left prefrontal rTMS. Patients completed a neuropsychological battery at baseline and after completing the protocol. Their preliminary findings suggest that rTMS may be an effective and safe treatment alternative for patients with refractory depression and stroke.

Emotional lability

Emotional lability following stroke can lead to difficulties in assessing mental state. The incidence is probably 15% following stroke (House *et al*, 1990; Andersen, 1995). It is characterised by the abrupt onset of weeping (or, more rarely, laughing), which is uncontrollable. There is often no obvious precipitant, although it can be triggered by emotion or emotional content — for example, on discussing home or seeing family members.

The symptoms themselves are usually distressing for the patient, family and also for ward staff. Emotional lability can also interfere with the rehabilitation process, delay progress and affect social functioning, and it is therefore important to diagnose and manage it appropriately (Andersen, 1995). Scales have been suggested and validated for the measurement of lability (Robinson *et al*, 1993; Brown *et al*, 1998). The aetiology of emotional lability is not known, although it does occur more often in patients with psychological symptoms and cognitive impairments. There is no proven correlation with lesion location, although it is postulated that damage to serotonergic transmission is important.

Emotional lability tends to improve over time, and explanation to the patient and family may be all that is required. Several studies have demonstrated the effectiveness of tricyclic antidepressants and SSRIs (Schiffer *et al*, 1985; Sloan *et al*, 1992; Robinson *et al*, 1993; Andersen, 1995; Brown *et al*, 1998), often with a rapid response to treatment (within one week). No evidence exists on optimal duration of therapy: this is another issue requiring further well-designed trials.

Conclusion

Depression following stroke is relatively common, perhaps affecting one in four hospitalised patients. Given that depression is known to correlate with poor outcome following stroke, all patients should have a screening assessment following stroke to identify the high-risk groups.

However, definite diagnosis of depression following stroke is not straightforward. Ideally, there would be a standard tool for use following stroke — but none are ideal. The HADS is well-studied and easy to administer; it may be the most appropriate tool if it can be further validated with standard thresholds for use following stroke. It may be that a diagnosis of PSD can never be certain, but treatment should be given on the likelihood of symptom response using a specified, validated assessment tool.

There is some evidence for effective treatments using nortryptiline and trazodone, but no large studies using the current commonly prescribed drugs, eg. fluoxetine, paroxetine and sertraline. Evidence suggests that treatment is of little benefit early (<6 weeks) after stroke. An initial monitoring and supportive role is appropriate, reserving medication for symptoms persisting after six weeks.

It is not yet known whether treatment reverses the poorer prognosis associated with PSD. This is another area worthy of further research, although it is unlikely to change our recommendations for increased awareness and treatment of this common, distressing and disabling disorder.

Post-stroke depression

References

Aben I, Denollet J, Lousberg R, Verhey F, Wojciechowski F, Honig A (2002) Personality and vulnerability to depression in stroke patients, a 1-year prospective follow-up study. *Stroke* **33**(10): 2391–5

Abiodun OA (1994) A validity study of the hospital anxiety and depression scale in general hospital units and a community hospital sample in Nigeria. *Br J Psychiatry* **165**: 669–72

Andersen G (1995) Treatment of uncontrolled crying after stroke. *Drugs Ageing* **16**: 105–11

Andersen G, Vestergaard K, Lauritzen L (1994) Effective treatment of post-stroke depression with the selective serotonin reuptake inhibitor citalopram. *Stroke* **25**: 1099–104

Astrom M, Adolfson R, Asplund K (1993) Major depression in stroke patients. *Stroke* **24**: 976–82

Beck AT, Ward CH, Mendelson M, Mock J, Erbaugh J (1961) An inventory for measuring depression. *Arch Gen Psychiatry* **4**: 53–63

Berg A, Palomaki H, Lethihalmes M, Lonnqvist J, Kaste M (2001) Post-stroke depression in acute phase after stroke. *Cerebrovasc Dis* **12**(1): 14–20

Berg A, Palomaki H, Lethihalmes M, Lonnqvist J, Kaste M (2003) Post-stroke depression: an 18-month follow-up. *Stroke* **34**(1): 138–43

Bridges KW, Goldberg DP (1986) The validation of the GHQ-28 and the use of the MMSE in neurological inpatients. *Br J Psychiatry* **148**: 548–53

Brown KW, Sloan RL, Pentland B (1998) Fluoxetine as a treatment for post-stroke emotionalism. *Acta Psychiat Scand* **6**: 455–8

Bryer JP, Starksein SE, Votypka V, Parikh RM, Price TR, Robinson RG (1992) Reduction of CSF monoamine metabolites in post-stroke depression: a preliminary report. *J Neuropsych Clin Neurosci* **4**: 440–2

Burvill JG, Anderson CS, Jamrozik K, Stewart-Wynne EG, Chakera TMH (1995) Screening instruments for depression and anxiety following stroke: experience in the Perth community stroke study. *Acta Psychiat Scand* **91**: 252–7

Cassidy E, O'Conner R, O' Keane V (2004) Prevalence of post-stroke depression in an Irish sample and its relationship with disability and outcome following inpatient rehabilitation. *Disabil Rehabil* **26**(2): 71–7

Clark MS, Smith DS (1998) The effects of depression and abnormal illness behaviour on outcome following rehabilitation from stroke. *Clin Rehabil* **12**: 73-80

Clark MS, Smith DS (1999) Psychological correlates of outcome following rehabilitation from stroke. *Clin Rehabil* 13: 129–40

Currier MB, Murray GB, Welch CC (1992) Electroconvulsive therapy for post-stroke depressed geriatric patients. *J Neuropsych Clin Neurosci* **4**: 140–4

Dahmen N, Marx J, Hops HC, Tettenborn B, Roder R (1999) Therapy of early post-stroke depression with venlafaxine: safety, tolerability and efficacy as determined in an open uncontrolled clinical trial. [Letter] *Stroke* **30**(3): 691–2

Dam M, Tonin P, De Boni A *et al* (1996) Effects of fluoxetine and maprotiline on functional recovery in post-stroke hemiplegic patients undergoing rehabilitation therapy. *Stroke* **27:** 1211–4

Davies B, Burrows G, Poynton C (1975) A comparative study of four depression rating scales. *Aust NZ J Psychiatry* **9:** 21–4

Dennis M, O'Rourke S, Slattery J, Staniforth T, Warlow C (1997) Evaluation of a stroke family care worker: results of a randomised controlled trial. *Br Med J* **314:** 1071–7

Drummond A, Walker M (1996) Generalization of the effects of leisure rehabilitation for stroke patients. *Br J Occup Ther* **59:** 330–4

Eriksson M, Asplund K, Glader EL, Norrving B, Stegmayr B, Terent A, Asberg KH, Wester PO (2004) Riks-Stroke Collaboration: self-reported depression and use of antidepressants after stroke: a national survey. *Stroke* **35**(4): 936–41

Everson SA, Roberts RE, Goldberg DE, Kaplan GA (1998) Depressive symptoms and increased risk of stroke mortality over a 29-year period. *Arch Intern Med* **158:** 1133–8

Folstein M, Maiberger R, McHugh P (1977) Mood disorder as a specific complication of stroke. *J Neurol Neurosurg Psychiatry* **40**: 1018–20

Fruehwald S, Gatterbauer E, Rehak P, Baumhackl U (2003) Early fluoxetine treatment of post-stroke depression: a three-month double-blind placebo-controlled study with an open-label long-term follow-up. *J Neurol* **250**(3): 347–51

Gainotti G, Antonucci G, Marra C, Paolucci S (2001) Relation between depression after stroke, antidepressant therapy and functional recovery. *J Neurol Neurosurg Psychiatry* **71**(2): 258–61

Gelder M, Gath D, Mayou R, Cowen P (1996) *Oxford Textbook of Psychiatry*. Oxford University Press, Oxford

Grade C, Redford B, Chrostowski J, Toussaint L, BlackwellB (1998) Methylphenidate in early post-stroke recovery: a double-blind placebo-controlled study. *Arch Phys Med Rehabil* **79**(9): 1047–50

Helzer JE (1983) Standardized interviews in psychiatry. *Psychiatr Dev* **1**(2): 161–78

Herrmann N, Black SE, Lawrence J, Szekely C, Szalai JP (1998) The Sunnybrook stroke study. *Stroke* **29:** 618–24

House A, Dennis M, Molyneux A, Warlow C, Haughton K (1990) Emotionalism after stroke. *Br Med J* **298:** 991–4

Jorge RE, Robinson RG, Tateno A, Narishima K, Acion L, Moser D, Ardnt S, Chemorinski E (2004) Repetitive transcranial magnetic stimulation as treatment of post-stroke depression: a preliminary study. *Biol Psychiatry* **55**(4): 398–405

Kimura M, Kanetani K, Imai R, Suzuki H, Isayama K, Endo S (2002) Therapeutic effects of milnacipran, a serotonin and noradrenaline reuptake inhibitor, on post-stroke depression. *Int Clin Psychopharmacol* **17**(3): 121–5

Kotila M, Numminen H, Waltimo O, Kaste M (1998) Depression after stroke: results of the FINNSTROKE study. *Stroke* **29:** 368–72

Lazarus LW, Moberg PJ, Langsley PR, Lingham VR (1994) Methylphenidate and nortriptyline in the treatment of post-stroke depression: a retrospective comparison. *Arch Phys Med*

Rehabil **75:** 403–6

Lesher EL, Berryhill JS (1994) Validation of the Geriatric Depression Scale-Short Form among inpatients. *J Clin Psychiatry* **50:** 256–60

Lincoln NB, Flannaghan T, Sutcliffe L, Rother L (1997) Evaluation of cognitive behavioural treatment for depression after stroke: a pilot study. *Clin Rehabil* **11:** 114–22

Lincoln NB, Flannagham T (2003) Cognitive behavioural psychotherapy for depression following stroke: a randomised controlled trial. *Stroke* **34**(1): 111–5

Lincoln NB, Nicholl CR, Flannagham T, Leonard M, Van der Gucht E (2003) The validity of questionnaire measures for assessing depression after stroke. *Clin Rehabil* **17**(8): 840–6

Lipsey JR, Pearlson GD, Price TR, Robinson RG, Rao K (1984) Nortriptyline treatment of post-stroke depression: a double-blind study. *Lancet* **i:** 297–300

Masand P, Murray G, Pickett P (1991) Psycho-stimulants in post-stroke depression. *J Neuropsych Clin Neurosci* **3:** 23–7

Montgomery S, Asberg M (1979) A new depression scale designed to be sensitive to change. *Br J Psychiatry* **134**: 322–89

Morris PLP, Raphael B, Robinson RG (1992) Clinical depression is associated with impaired recovery from stroke. *Med J Aust* **157:** 239–42

Morris P, Hopwood M, Maguire K, Norman T, Schweitzer I (2003) Blunted prolactin response to D-fenfluramine in post-stroke major depression. *J Affect Disord* **76**(1–3): 273–8

Murray GB, Shea VM, Conn DK (1986) Electroconvulsive therapy for post-stroke depression. *J Clin Psychiatry* **47**: 258–60

Narushima K, Kosier JT, Robinson RG (2002) Preventing post-stroke depression: a 12 week double-blind randomised treatment trial and 21 month follow-up. *J Nerv Ment Dis* **190**(5): 296–303

O'Rourke S, MacHale S, Signorini D, Dennis M (1998) Detecting psychiatric morbidity after stroke: comparison of the GHQ and the HAD scale. *Stroke* **29:** 980–5

Palomaki H, Kaste M, Berg A, Lonnqvist J, Lonnqvist J, Lehtihmes M, Hares J (1999) Prevention of post-stroke depression: 1 year randomised placebo-controlled double-blind trial of mianserin with 6 month follow up after therapy. *J Neurol Neurosurg Psychiatry* **66**(4): 490–4

Paolucci S, Antonucci G, Grasso MG, Morelli D, Troisi E, Coiro P, De Angelis D, Rizzi F, Bragoni M (2001) Post-stroke depression, antidepressant treatment and rehabilitation: a case-control study. *Cerebrovasc Dis* **12**(3): 264–71

Pohjasvaara T, Leppavuori A, Siira I, Vataja R, Kaste M, Erkinjuntti T (1998) Frequency and clinical determinants of post-stroke depression. *Stroke* **29:** 2311–7

Pohjasvaara T, Vataja R, Leppavuori A, Kaste M, Erkinjuntti T (2001) Depression is an independent predictor of poor long-term functional outcome post-stroke. *Eur J Neurol* **8**(4): 315–9

Ramasubbu R, Flint A, Brown G, Awad G, Kennedy S (1998) Diminished serotonin-mediated prolactin responses in non-depressed stroke patients compared with healthy normal subjects. *Stroke* **29:** 1293–8

Rasmussen A, Lunde M, Poulsen DL, Sorensen K, Qvitzau S, Bech P (2003) A double-blind, placebo-controlled study of sertaline in the prevention of depression in stroke patients. [Erratum appears in *Psychosomatics* (2004) Jan-Feb **45**(1): 91]. *Psychosomatics* **44**(3): 216–21

Reding MJ, Orto LA, Winter SW, Fortuna IM, Ponte PD, McDowell FH (1986) Antidepressant therapy after stroke: a double-blind trial. *Arch Neurol* **43**: 763–5

Robinson RG, Parikh RM, Lipsey JR, Starkstein SE, Price TR (1993) Pathological laughing and crying following stroke — validation of a measurement scale and a double-blind treatment study. *Am J Psychiatry* **150**: 286–93

Schiffer RB, Herndon RM, Rudick RA (1985) Treatment of pathological laughing and weeping with amitryptilline. *N Engl J Med* **314**: 1480–2

Sloan RL, Brown KW, Pentland B (1992) Fluoxetine as a treatment for emotional lability after brain injury. *Brain Injury* **6**: 315–9

Spinhoven PH, Ormal J, Sloekers PPA, Kempen GIJM, Speckens AEM, Van Hemert AM (1997) A validation study of the Hospital Anxiety and Depression Scale in different groups of Dutch subjects. *Psychol Med* **27**: 363–70

Stenager EN, Madsen C, Stenager E, Boldsen J (1998) Suicide in patients with stroke: epidemiological study. *Br Med J* **316**: 1206

Sutcliffe L, Lincoln N (1998) The assessment of depression in aphasic stroke patients: the development of the Stroke Aphasic Depression Questionnaire. *Clin Rehabil* **12**: 506–13

Turner-Stokes L, Hassan N (2002) Depression after stroke: a review of the evidence-base to inform the development of an integrated care pathway. Part 1: Diagnosis, frequency and impact. [Review] [94 refs]. *Clin Rehabil* **16**(3): 231–47

Verdello A, Henon H, Lebert F, Pasquier F, Leys D (2004) Depressive symptoms after stroke and relationship with dementia: a three-year follow-up study. *Neurology* **62**(6): 905–11

Wade D (1992) Stroke: rehabilitation and long-term care. *Lancet* **339**: 791–3

Wade DT, Legh-Smith J, Hewer RA (1987) Depressed mood after stroke: a community study of its frequency. *Br J Psychiatry* **151**: 200–5

Yesavage JA, Brink TL, Rose TL, Lum O, Haung Z, Adey M, Leirer VO (1982–83) Development and validation of a geriatric depression screening scale: a preliminary report. *J Psychiatr Res* **17**: 37–49

Zifko UA, Rupp M, Schwarz S (2002) [Sertaline in the treatment of post-stroke depression results of an open multicentre study] [German]. *Wien Med Wochensch* **152**(13–14): 343–8

Zigmond A, Snaith R (1983) The Hospital Anxiety and Depression Scale. *Acta Psychiatr Scand* **67**: 364–70

CHAPTER 10

Assessment and management of dysphagia

Deborah JC Ramsey, David G Smithard

Swallowing problems are common in hospital inpatients and may affect morbidity and mortality. Accurate assessment of dysphagia is important, allowing optimal management and minimising potential complications. This chapter considers the methods of swallow assessment and ways in which problems can be addressed.

Swallowing (*Figure 10.1*) is a complex procedure involving the use of six cranial nerves and fifty-five muscles (Smithard, 2002a; Diamant, 1995). It consists of three phases: oral, pharyngeal and oesophageal. Apart from the first part of the oral phase, which is under voluntary control, swallowing is predominantly an involuntary process, the stages of which are modified by the

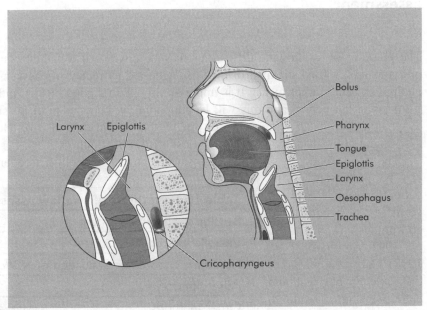

Figure 10.1: Principal structures involved in swallowing

characteristics of the bolus and by input from higher cortical and subcortical centres (*Figure 10.2*). A safe swallow requires coordination such that the sequential phases are in synchrony not only with each other but also with respiration, since respiration must cease as swallowing commences to allow concomitant airway protection; exhalation then occurs when the swallow is complete.

Difficulty in swallowing (dysphagia) is common in many acute and chronic neurological conditions (eg. stroke), head and neck disease, and oesophageal disorders (Logemann, 1995). As well as causing psychological distress, dysphagia may increase morbidity and mortality (Smithard *et al*, 1996). Many patients with abnormal swallowing are at risk of aspiration (the passage of food or fluid below the true vocal cords) and its associated morbidity (Schmidt *et al*, 1994). This chapter reviews the various methods of oropharyngeal swallow assessment that are available (*Table 10.1*) and then considers practical points in the management of a dysphagic patient.

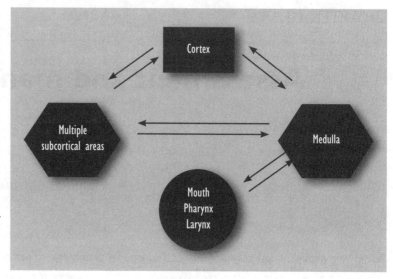

Figure 10.2: A diagrammatic representation of the complex neurological control of swallowing

Bedside swallow assessment

The presence of swallowing difficulties may be obvious if a patient coughs during oral intake or complains of food sticking, or may be suggested by recurrent chest infections or a wet voice quality, especially after meals. It is important to obtain a good history, either from the patient or from his or her carers, and this will be supported by knowledge of possible aetiologies for the dysphagia, such as an acute stroke or progressive Parkinson's disease. However, a more formal assessment of the swallow itself will almost always be required.

The term 'bedside swallow assessment' covers several heterogeneous techniques that can be performed at the patient's bedside without significant additional equipment (Linden *et al*, 1993; Smithard *et al*, 1998). General appraisal of the patient's physical and cognitive state is required, and most methods involve an assessment of oromotor function, including tongue function, facial weakness, ability to produce a voluntary cough and voice quality. The gag reflex has traditionally been tested as an indicator of swallow

Table 10.1: Methods of swallow assessment

Bedside swallow assessment	
Videofluoroscopy	
Fibreoptic endoscopic evaluation of swallowing	
Pulse oximetry	
Other methods	Cervical auscultation
	Lateral cervical soft tissue radiography post contrast
	Ultrasonography
	Pharyngeal or oesophageal manometry
	Scintigraphy
	Electromyography

function, but many studies have failed to find a convincing link between an absent gag and dysphagia (Smithard *et al*, 1998; McCullough *et al*, 2001). A gag reflex may be absent in a significant proportion of healthy adults (Davies *et al*, 1995), and the differing neurological basis of the gag reflex and the swallow mechanism makes it unsurprising that the two are not clearly linked (Logemann, 1995).

Following an initial assessment, patients are challenged with food or fluid, usually starting with small volumes of water in case of difficulty and then trying other volumes of food and liquid. The degree of laryngeal elevation is noted, as is the amount of effort required to swallow, and patients are observed for coughing, signs of respiratory distress and any change in voice quality. Some swallow assessments include additional features such as the time required to swallow a set volume of liquid (Hinds and Wiles, 1998), the latent time to swallowing (Teramoto and Fukuchi, 2000), or the presence or absence of an adequate laryngeal cough reflex (Addington *et al*, 1999). Other workers have assessed laryngopharyngeal sensation by directing air pulses at the mucosa supplied by the superior laryngeal nerve (Aviv *et al*, 1998).

Although bedside swallow assessments are practical in a clinical setting, being possible in most patients who are alert enough to feed even if they are too ill to leave the ward, they have limitations. Validity studies using videofluoroscopy (VF) for comparison have found wide-ranging sensitivity, specificity and predictive values for these tests (Splaingard *et al*, 1988; Smithard *et al*, 1998; Smith *et al*, 2000). For example, the phenomenon of silent aspiration, in which aspiration occurs without coughing or other outward sign of difficulty (Horner and Massey, 1988), is by definition difficult to detect at the bedside. In addition, inter- and intra-rater reliability for these assessments may be very poor (Smithard *et al*, 1998; McCullough *et al*, 2000).

Videofluoroscopy (VF)

Videofluoroscopy (VF) or modified barium swallow is regarded by many as the method of choice in assessing swallowing (O'Donoghue and Bagnall, 1999). It involves imaging a patient sitting at 45–90° while he or she swallows food or fluids of different consistencies which have been impregnated with contrast agent (usually barium). The technique allows real-time visualisation of the structural and functional elements of swallowing, as well as testing of potential compensatory techniques (Logemann, 1995).

VF provides a dynamic assessment of swallowing but has logistical disadvantages (Ramsey *et al*, 2003). Not all hospitals offer the procedure, which requires a patient to be able to sit relatively upright and be well enough to leave the ward. The test provides a brief snapshot of the patient's swallowing in a well-supervised environment which may not be representative of their time on the ward, and does not take into account swallow fatigue during a meal prolonged by dysphagia. The radiation exposure involved makes the study inappropriate for frequent repetition, but repeat trials of each consistency are required within a session, since test–test variability within patients has been described (Lof and Robbins, 1990). Inter-rater reliability for interpretation of a study is variable, but probably better with training and experience (Ekberg *et al*, 1988).

Fibreoptic endoscopic evaluation of swallowing (FEES)

Fibreoptic endoscopic evaluation of swallowing (FEES) is used in some centres to visualise local anatomy and the swallow process itself (Aviv et al, 1998). Aspiration cannot be seen directly because of the 'white-out' during swallowing, but may be inferred from residue left afterwards or from the sight of food being ejected from the trachea. The procedure is safe and generally well-tolerated (Aviv et al, 2000) and may be performed at the bedside and recorded for later review. However, it requires a trained operator and specialist equipment and is not available in all centres. Comparison with VF and with outcomes suggests it is a valid procedure (Langmore et al, 1991).

Pulse oximetry

A number of studies have suggested that desaturation on pulse oximetry during swallowing may serve as a marker of aspiration (Zaidi et al, 1995; Collins and Bakheit, 1997; Smith et al, 2000), either by reflex bronchoconstriction or via a poor breathing pattern while swallowing (Zaidi et al, 1995; Teramoto et al, 1996). Although not all studies confirm the association (Colodny, 2000), comparisons of saturations with VF or FEES have given reasonable sensitivities and specificities (Collins and Bakheit, 1997; Smith et al, 2000; Lim et al, 2001); using aspiration or penetration as the end point rather than aspiration alone was more predictive (Smith et al, 2000). Use of saturation data in combination with a bedside clinical assessment may be more useful than in isolation (Smith et al, 2000; Lim et al, 2001), but further work is required before pulse oximetry can be part of routine assessment.

Other methods

Various other methods of swallow testing have been used but primarily only as research tools. These include cervical auscultation (Zenner et al, 1995); lateral cervical soft tissue radiography after contrast swallowing (Bradford et al, 2000); ultrasonography (Smithard, 2002b); pharyngeal or oesophageal manometry (Hila et al, 2001); scintigraphy (Muz et al, 1991); and electromyography (Palmer et al, 1992).

Management of dysphagia

Once a diagnosis of dysphagia has been made, effective management (*Table 10.2*) comprises two main components: prevention of aspiration and maintenance of adequate nutritional intake. Any assessment must first determine whether a person is alert and well enough to try swallowing. Patients with a significantly depressed conscious level cannot protect their airway against aspiration of their own saliva, making oral feeding wholly inappropriate. Other individuals may be alert for short periods but then become fatigued, putting them at risk of aspiration with a prolonged meal. An individual's level of attention is also important: a tendency to distraction may lead to an attempt to speak while swallowing, leaving the airway unprotected. Swallowing must always be performed with a patient in the most upright position possible to optimise swallow safety. In addition, to be able to follow and benefit from interventions, a patient must be aware of their swallowing problems; the more aware they are, the less likely they are to develop secondary complications (Parker *et al*, 2004).

If oral intake is appropriate, several strategies (*Table 10.3*) are available to assist in safe swallowing. Postural techniques and compensatory manoeuvres may be used in dysphagic patients who can follow instructions (Logemann, 1995); for example, in patients with unilateral pharyngeal paresis, turning the head towards the damaged side while swallowing may help prevent passage of food down the damaged side of the oropharynx, minimising aspiration from residue which might otherwise collect on this side. Tucking the chin down may help patients in whom posterior movement of the tongue base is impaired by pushing food back towards the pharyngeal wall. The manoeuvre also narrows the laryngeal entrance somewhat, reducing the risk of aspiration if triggering of the swallow is delayed.

Table 10.2: Management considerations in dysphagic patients

Level of alertness
Cognition
Posture and compensatory techniques (eg. head turning)
Consistency of fluids
Volume of fluids
Supervision of meals
Swallow exercises
Increased sensory input
Nasogastric feeding
Percutaneous endoscopic gastrostomy feeding (PEG)

Table 10.3: Strategies to aid in the management of oropharyngeal dysphagia

Disorder		Postural technique	Appropriate food consistencies
Oral stage	Reduced cheek tension	Tilt head to stronger side	Thin liquid to pureed
	Reduced tongue elevation	Tilt head back	Thin to thick liquids
Triggering of pharyngeal swallow	Delayed/absent	Chin down	Avoid thin liquids
Pharyngeal stage	Unilateral pharyngeal weakness	Rotate head to weaker side	Liquids to thin pureed
	Bilateral pharyngeal weakness	Lie down	Liquids to thin pureed
	Reduced laryngeal elevation	Chin down	Thick liquid to solid food

Other manoeuvres can be used in patients able to understand more complex instructions, such as the supraglottic swallow, in which the true vocal folds are closed before and during the swallow via use of a voluntary breath hold; this may be of help in patients with reduced or late vocal fold closure and a delayed pharyngeal swallow.

Whether or not postural measures are successful, changing the consistency and type of food or fluid for different individuals may be of help (*Table 10.3*). Simple measures such as cutting up food may alleviate difficulties for patients with a paretic hand. Supervised meals may allow safe feeding in individuals who tend to distraction or fatigue. Small volumes such as sips or teaspoonfuls may be easier to manage than larger ones. In terms of consistency, thin liquids such as water may be less likely to cause physical obstruction of the airway but can be difficult to maintain as a cohesive bolus in the oropharynx if there are problems such as facial or tongue weakness; thicker consistencies may be easier. However, thin liquids would be inappropriate in individuals in whom swallow triggering is delayed or absent, since they may easily fall backwards into the open airway.

Some patients may benefit from swallow exercises, for example, to improve the activity of the base of the tongue and the pharyngeal wall after head and neck surgery (Logemann, 1995). In other individuals, techniques may be tried to increase local sensory input before swallowing (Logemann, 1995; Smithard, 1995) in the hope that this may alert the CNS to the presence of a bolus to be swallowed. For example, a bolus may be used with a strong (perhaps sour) flavour, or increased tactile pressure may be applied in the oral cavity or the anterior faucial arches with a spoon or cold laryngeal mirror before an attempt to swallow.

It should be acknowledged that the evidence-base for the use of a cold thermal stimulus at the base of the faucial pillars is weak. De Lama Lazzara *et al* (1986) reported benefits using a cold 00 laryngeal mirror but the population group was of mixed disease processes. Hamdy *et al* (2003) found that a cold-water stimulus did not affect the swallow significantly, but that cold water with 5mls of 10% lemon juice added actually prolonged the swallow and people took smaller sips less frequently. They suggested that the heightened sensory input from both cold and lemon juice produced a stimulus that may have been noxious and surmised that the smaller swallows may be protective. This seems to be supported by Fraser *et al* (2002) who noted that low-frequency electrical stimulation of the pharynx facilitated corticobulbar excitability, whereas higher frequencies had an inhibitory effect. Corticobulbar plasticity also seems to have functionally relevant effects on aspiration.

Others have tried to use electrical stimulation, either to the palate (Park *et al*, 1997) or transcutaneously to the pharyngeal region via electrodes on the neck (Vitastim) (Freed *et al*, 2001). Both studies are small and consequently need further work. Vitastim has been approved by the US Food and Drugs Administration following collection of five years' worth of data.

A number of patients are assessed as completely unsafe to swallow. A transient period of support via intravenous fluids may be appropriate (for example, in patients who are drowsy following a general anaesthetic). However, after twenty-four to forty-eight hours of no swallowing, enteral feeding should be considered to minimise malnutrition and discomfort for the patient. Initial support in dysphagic patients generally involves feeding through a nasogastric tube, which may also be used in patients who can swallow small amounts safely but are unable to manage sufficient orally to support their nutritional requirements. Patients with prolonged severe dysphagia or those who are finding it difficult to tolerate a nasogastric tube should be considered for insertion of a percutaneous endoscopic gastrostomy (PEG) tube. This is a more invasive procedure with associated morbidity and mortality (Pennington, 2002) and does not prevent aspiration of a patient's own secretions, although it does allow maintenance of nutrition.

The release of the FOOD trial results (reported during the European Stroke Conference, Mannheim, Germany, May 2004) sheds some important light on the effectiveness of enteral and sip feeding. The results suggest that early nasogastric feeding may have a positive effect on reducing poor outcome, although the confidence intervals are wide. The early placement of a PEG tube does not affect outcome. The use of supplements was also unproven.

Ethical issues

It is important for care-providers to recognise that persistent failure to eat will result in death, as well as prolonging recovery from illness and predisposing to malnutrition-associated problems such as pressure ulcers and infections. Access to food and fluid is a basic human right for all individuals expressing a desire to eat or drink, and these should be provided in the absence of medical contraindications. However, a competent adult has the legal right to refuse a treatment should they wish to do so (Lennard-Jones, 1999) and indeed perceptions of quality of life may vary between individuals, with some patients finding severe debility relatively acceptable and others considering less severe illness as intolerable, undignified suffering. In the USA, laws now exist to ensure that previously stated patient preferences regarding medical treatments and life-sustaining treatments are honoured, and similar recognition of such documents is advised in the UK as well.

Ethical issues may arise in the care of persons without the mental competence to make clear their wishes, particularly if food or fluids would need to be provided via artificial means. In England and Wales, another person cannot give consent on behalf of a mentally incapable adult (Lennard-Jones, 1999) and decisions for such individuals are the responsibility of the medical and mutidisciplinary team involved, acting in the best interests of the patient, seeking any previously expressed wishes on such treatments from family and carers if possible.

In recent years in the UK, there has been much debate regarding the provision of nutrition to patients with severe brain injury, terminal disease (eg. metastatic malignancy) or end-stage dementia. A balance needs to be achieved between the prevention of untimely death and the postponement of the inevitable. In some situations the decisions are simple, but ethical and moral dilemmas may arise for patients who are neither dying nor clearly improving. In some circumstances, it may be appropriate to use enteral nutrition as a palliative tool rather than as a curative treatment.

Currently, in UK law, tube feeding is regarded as a medical treatment rather than as basic mandatory care (Lennard-Jones, 1999), and it can therefore be withheld or withdrawn if this is felt appropriate by the medical team responsible. However, in this situation, it is important for a patient's loved ones to be aware that withholding or withdrawing tube feeding does not mean withdrawal of all treatment. All patients must be offered whatever care is necessary to relieve any pain and suffering, and it should be made clear that death from dehydration is generally a peaceful, pain-free death (increased potassium levels, ketones and endorphins). If providing nutrition is felt to be appropriate, the cost/benefit (burden) ratio for the patient needs to be considered. It may be felt appropriate to start treatment as a time-limited trial, to be reviewed at the end of a specified time, but withdrawal of therapy is emotionally more difficult than withholding it and it is difficult to know how to assess the success of a short period of nutritional support. Dyer (2004) reported on a man with degenerative cerebellar ataxia who challenged the guidance issued by the General Medical Council (GMC), which had suggested that medical staff should make decisions on whether or not to feed and, in particular, could decide to withdraw if the situation appears futile. The challenge was upheld, but there may be an appeal by the GMC before guidance is changed.

Consent for the provision of enteral nutrition is often assumed to have been given in the passing of a nasogastric tube, unless insertion is actively resisted. Repeated subsequent removals of nasogastric tubes may mean refusal of nutrition or may simply reflect discomfort from a local irritant. The insertion of a PEG tube, a more invasive procedure, requires formal informed consent and this may be difficult to obtain, especially in a dysphasic, cognitively impaired or acutely confused patient, making it the responsibility of the treating doctor. Questions remain as to what is in the best interest of the patient, what is quality of life, whose quality of life and also as to whether in reality we are treating a patient, his or her family, or ourselves (Smithard, 1999). Whatever decision is made, it must be made after consultation with the relatives and the multidisciplinary team so that all are aware of any decision to feed or not to feed, as failure to supply fluids and food will ultimately result in death.

Conclusions

Swallowing problems are common in an inpatient setting and may present significant challenges to the staff involved. A number of methods of assessment are available depending on a unit's resources, although the most commonly used test in most places is still the bedside assessment. VF is often the next method used but this and other more complex techniques all have their limitations. Once diagnosed, dysphagia may be managed via a number of strategies depending on the patient and the underlying cause of the dysphagia. The importance of effective and appropriate management of these problems is highlighted by the potential for increased morbidity and mortality in dysphagic patients. Ethical issues in the nutritional support of dysphagic patients unable to express their own wishes directly can be challenging.

Figure 10.1 is adapted from Smithard (1995).

References

Addington WR, Stephens RE, Gilliland K, Rodriguez M (1999) Assessing the laryngeal cough reflex and the risk of developing pneumonia after stroke. *Arch Phys Med Rehabil* **80**: 150–4

Aviv JE, Kim T, Sacco RL, Kaplan S, Goodhart K, Diamond B, Close LG (1998) FEESST: a new bedside endoscopic test of the motor and sensory components of swallowing. *Ann Otol Rhinol Laryngol* **107**: 378–87

Aviv JE, Kaplan ST, Thomson JE, Spitzer J, Diamond B, Close LG (2000) The safety of flexible endoscopic evaluation of swallowing with sensory testing (FEESST): an analysis of 500 consecutive evaluations. *Dysphagia* **15**(1): 39–44

Bradford APJ, Begg T, Adams FG, Lees KR (2000) Post stroke aspiration risk assessment using a contrast lateral cervical soft tissue X-ray. Presentation at British Association of Stroke Physicians Annual Conference, Liverpool, UK

Collins MJ, Bakheit AMO (1997) Does pulse oximetry reliably detect aspiration in dysphagic stroke patients? *Stroke* **28**(9): 1773–5

Colodny N (2000) Comparison of dysphagics and nondysphagics on pulse oximetry during oral feeding. *Dysphagia* **15**(2): 68–73

Davies AE, Kidd D, Stone SP, MacMahon J (1995) Pharyngeal sensation and gag reflex in healthy subjects. *Lancet* **345**: 487–8

De Lama Lazzara G, Lazarus C, Logemann JA (1986) Impact of thermal stimulation on the triggering of the swallowing reflex. *Dysphagia* **1**(2): 73–7

Diamant NE (1995) A glimpse at the central mechanism for swallowing. *Gastroenterol* **109**: 1700–02

Dyer O (2004) Man wins battle to keep receiving life support. *BMJ* **329**(7461): 309

Ekberg O, Nylander G, Fork F, Sjoberg S, Birch-Iensen M, Hillarp B (1988) Interobserver variability in cineradiographic assessment of pharyngeal function during swallow. *Dysphagia* **3**: 46–8

Fraser C, Power M, Hamdy S, *et al* (2002) Driving plasticity in human adult motor cortex is associated with improved motor function after brain injury. *Neuron* **34**: 831–40

Freed ML, Freed L, Chatburn RL, *et al* (2001) Electrical stimulation for swallowing disorders caused by stroke. *Respiratory Care* **46**(5): 466–74

Hamdy S, Jilani S, Price V, *et al* (2003) Modulation of human swallowing behaviour by thermal and chemical stimulation in health and after brain injury. *Neurogastroenterol Motil* **15**: 69–77

Hila A, Castell JA, Castell DO (2001) Pharyngeal and upper esophageal sphincter manometry in the evaluation of dysphagia. *J Clin Gastroenterol* **33**(5): 355–61

Hinds NP, Wiles CM (1998) Assessment of swallowing and referral to speech and language therapists in acute stroke. *QJM* **91**: 829–35

Horner J, Massey EW (1988) Silent aspiration following stroke. *Neurology* **38**(2): 317–19

Langmore SE, Schatz K, Olson N (1991) Endoscopic and videofluoroscopic evaluations of swallowing and aspiration. *Ann Otol Laryngol* **100**: 678–81

Lennard-Jones JE (1999) Giving or withholding fluid and nutrients: ethical and legal aspects. *J R Coll Physicians Lond* **33**(1): 39–45

Lim SHB, Lieu PK, Phua SY, Seshadri R, Venketasubramanian N, Lee SH, Choo PWJ (2001) Accuracy of bedside clinical methods compared with fiberoptic endoscopic examination of swallowing (FEES) in determining the risk of aspiration in acute stroke patients. *Dysphagia* **16**(1): 1–6

Linden P, Kuhlemeier KV, Patterson C (1993) The probability of correctly predicting subglottic penetration from clinical observations. *Dysphagia* **8**(3): 170–9

Lof GL, Robbins J (1990) Test-retest variability in normal swallowing. *Dysphagia* **4**: 236–42

Logemann JA (1995) Dysphagia: evaluation and treatment. *Folia Phoniatr Logop* **47**: 140–64

McCullough GH, Wertz RT, Rosenbek JC, Mills RH, Ross KB, Ashford JR (2000) Inter- and intrajudge reliability of a clinical examination of swallowing in adults. *Dysphagia* **15**(2): 58–67

McCullough GH, Wertz RT, Rosenbek JC (2001) Sensitivity and specificity of clinical/bedside examination signs for detecting aspiration in adults subsequent to stroke. *J Commun Disord* **34**: 55–72

Muz J, Mathog RH, Hamlet SL, Davis LP, Kling GA (1991) Objective assessment of swallowing function in head and neck cancer patients. *Head Neck* **13**: 33–9

O'Donoghue S, Bagnall A (1999) Videofluoroscopic evaluation in the assessment of swallowing disorders in paediatric and adult populations. *Folia Phoniatr Logop* **51**: 158–71

Palmer JB, Rudin NJ, Lara G, Crompton AW (1992) Coordination of mastication and swallowing. *Dysphagia* **7**(4): 187–200

Park CL, O'Neill PA, Martin DF (1997) A pilot exploratory study of oral electrical stimulation on swallow function following stroke: an innovative tecnique. *Dysphagia* **12**(3): 161–66

Parker C, Power M, Hamdy S, *et al* (2004) Awareness of dysphagia by patients following stroke predicts swallowing performance. *Dysphagia* **19**(1): 28–35

Pennington C (2002) To PEG or not to PEG. *Clin Med JRCPL* **2**: 250–5

Ramsey DJC, Smithard DG, Kalra L (2003) Early assessments of dysphagia and aspiration risk in acute stroke patients. *Stroke* **34**(5): 1252–7

Schmidt J, Holas M, Halvorson K, Reding M (1994) Videofluoroscopic evidence of aspiration predicts pneumonia and death but not dehydration following stroke. *Dysphagia* **9**: 7–11

Smith HA, Lee SH, O'Neill PA, Connolly MJ (2000) The combination of bedside swallowing assessment and oxygen saturation monitoring of swallowing in acute stroke: a safe and humane screening tool. *Age Ageing* **29**: 495–9

Smithard DG (1995) Dysphagia assessment after acute stroke. *Hosp Update* **Dec**: 555–61

Smithard DG (1999) Dysphagia following stroke. *Rev Clin Geront* **9**: 81–93

Smithard DG (2002a) Swallowing and stroke. *Cerebrovasc Dis* **14**: 1–8

Smithard DG (2002b) Assessment of swallowing following stroke. *Stroke Review* **6**(2): 7–10

Smithard DG, O'Neill PA, Park C, Morris J, Wyatt R, England R, Martin DF (1996) Complications and outcome after acute stroke: does dysphagia matter? *Stroke* **27**(7): 1200–4

Smithard DG, O'Neill PA, Park C *et al* (1998) Can bedside assessment reliably exclude aspiration following acute stroke? *Age Ageing* **27**: 99–106

Splaingard ML, Hutchins B, Sulton LD, Chaudhuri G (1988) Aspiration in rehabilitation patients: videofluoroscopy *vs* bedside clinical assessment. *Arch Phys Med Rehabil* **69**: 637–40

Teramoto S, Fukuchi Y (2000) Detection of aspiration and swallowing disorder in older stroke patients: simple swallowing provocation test versus water swallowing test. *Arch Phys Med*

Rehabil **81**(11): 1517–19

Teramoto S, Fukuchi Y, Ouchi Y (1996) Oxygen desaturation on swallowing in patients with stroke: what does it mean? *Age Ageing* **25**: 333–6

Zaidi NH, Smith HA, King SC, Park C, O'Neill PA, Connolly MJ (1995) Oxygen desaturation on swallowing as a potential marker of aspiration in acute stroke. *Age Ageing* **24**: 267–70

Zenner PM, Losinski DS, Mills RH (1995) Using cervical auscultation in the clinical dysphagia examination in long-term care. *Dysphagia* **10**(1): 27–31

CHAPTER 11

Research in practice: management of swallowing difficulties post stroke

Ruth A Sullivan, Lynn K Dangerfield

This chapter presents a pilot study carried out in the workplace in order to shape future research into dysphagia after stroke. The authors looked at the clinical effectiveness of direct and indirect speech and language therapy in older patients with a stroke. The results were inconclusive, but they should provide a valuable lead for a full-scale study.

Stroke and dysphagia

It is estimated that up to 67% of people sustaining either a first or subsequent stroke will have some degree of swallowing difficulty (Hinds and Wiles, 1998). A high proportion of these resolve fairly quickly — about 50% within the first seven days and 75% within one month (Smithard *et al*, 1997). A brainstem stroke or lateral medullary syndrome and/or a history of previous strokes will almost certainly lengthen the recovery time.

Studies have shown that there is bilateral cortical representation of pharyngeal involvement and that there is some compensation in the unaffected hemisphere during recovery (Hamdy *et al*, 1998). In addition, both research evidence and working knowledge suggest a fairly predictable pattern of recovery following a single hemisphere stroke (Smithard *et al*, 1997).

Timely screening and appropriate management of swallowing difficulties are vital in order to minimise the risk of aspiration. Aspiration is a well-documented risk factor (Langmore, 1998) and is defined as the misdirection of oropharyngeal contents into the airway due to incoordination of the swallow process. In healthy individuals, such misdirection usually results in a cough to expel the food or fluid. In the older person, whose strength of cough may be weakened by the ageing process (Patteson, 1996; Nilsson *et al*, 1996) in addition to neurological damage resulting from a stroke and associated reduction in mobility, aspiration may not be tolerated. This puts the person at increased risk of chest infection.

The other major risk factor in management of this client group is malnutrition, with its well-documented effect on recovery and rehabilitation in terms of its effect on muscle tone and also on mood and motivation (Davilos, 1996; Gariballa, 1998; Perry, 2001). Furthermore, the nutritional status of many older people may be compromised pre-admission and studies have shown that in the non-dysphagic population there is a risk of weight loss following a hospital stay (McWhirter Pennington, 1994). *The Essence of Care Resource Pack* (2001) was developed to highlight nutritional issues within this population

To avoid any compromise in nutritional status for this client group, it is important to identify any associated dysphagia at the earliest opportunity.

The role of the nurse

The need for a combined approach to the assessment and management of dysphagia is well-documented in the literature. A logical and consistent approach from all relevant medical, nursing and therapy teams is vital (Perry, 2001). There is much evidence to indicate that appropriately trained nurses can manage dysphagia post-stroke with the support of speech and language therapy (Travers, 1999; Perry, 2001). An ENB publication (2001) examines the role and contribution of nurses within the multidisciplinary rehabilitation team and identifies that nurses are interested in a greater involvement and responsibility regarding swallowing assessment and management. As the main providers of twenty-four-hour care in the acute stages of dysphagia, it is appropriate that nurses are actively involved in dysphagia management. Screening tools may identify those at risk and assist nursing staff in this vital role. Examples include the Burke Dysphagia Screening Test (1994) and Standardised Swallow Assessment (SSA) (Ellul *et al*, 1997) and Bedside swallow assessment (Smithard *et al*, 1998). These all use water for the initial screen. The authors have developed screening tests further to produce functional dysphagia screening and management flowcharts that were used in this study (*Figures 11.1* and *11.2*). It is felt that these are more suited to both an older population and for those with stroke-induced dysphagia. In contrast to the above screening tools, the Portsmouth Dysphagia Flowcharts (DFC) use a range of consistencies from thickened /smooth to thin (Dangerfield and Sullivan, 1999). Since the project, these were revised in 2003 to incorporate the National Descriptors for Texture Modification (2003), developed as collaboration between the Royal College of Speech and Language Therapists (RCSLT) and the British Dietetics Association (BDA).

Dysphagia training for nursing staff

Educating those caring for people with dysphagia is a priority if these vital team members are to carry out the recommendations safely. Speech and language therapists (SLTs) have been involved in providing dysphagia training for nursing staff for several years, and this has a high profile within the hospital and community health settings in Portsmouth (UK). The dysphagia flowcharts are an integral part of this training and are well-received by trained nursing staff. The *National Service Framework for Older People* (DoH, 2001) highlights the need for providing person-focused care,

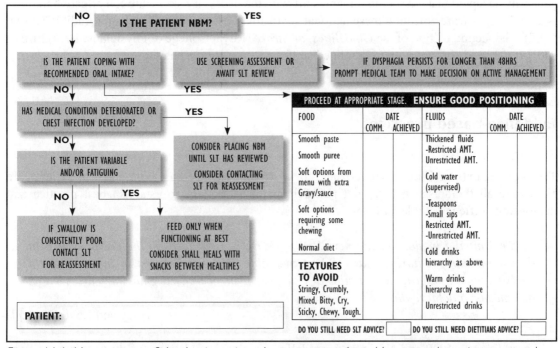

Figure 11.1: Management of dysphagic patients known to speech and language therapist — care plan

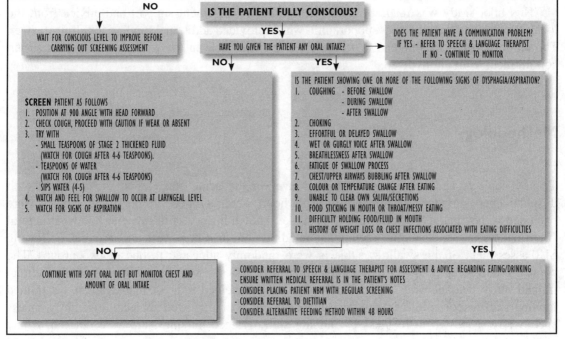

Figure 11.2: Screening assessment for dysphagic patients

promoting older persons' health and independence, and fitting services around peoples needs. It is generally accepted that equipping nursing staff with the necessary skills through effective training is a vital step towards meeting these national standards (Collaborative Dysphagia Audit [CODA], 1997). The second edition of the *Guidelines for Stroke* (Royal College of Physicians, 2004) further support the need for 'appropriately trained staff' to screen for dysphagia.

Evidence-based practice

The requirements of Clinical Governance for a strong evidence-based approach to patient care encourage all therapists to carry out research in the workplace to establish best practice and demonstrate efficacy at a local level.

> *In the United Kingdom in the new NHS, quality is envisaged as the driving force in decision-making requiring that the best available evidence be used to inform clinical decision-making and underpin clinical practice. Evidence-based guidelines are seen as one means to achieve this.*

Perry and Love (2001: 7)

In addition to RCP and NSF stroke guidelines, national guidelines for dysphagia have been produced by the RCSLT (2003). Local dysphagia guidelines have also been developed and audited; a system to ensure that they are regularly updated has also been established (CPOL Conference, 2003).

This pilot study was made possible with strong management support and advice from the local research and development support unit, which provided additional funding for clinical cover. The authors would recommend that any research sustainable in the workplace demands strong commitment from all involved.

Methodology

Twenty subjects aged sixty-five years and over in the acute stage of stroke recovery with dysphagia persisting for longer than forty-eight hours were recruited into the study. Subjects were excluded if they had a history of previous stroke; known history of dysphagia; known structural abnormality; known dementia; pneumonia on admission; or if they were unconscious. Following SLT assessment of the swallow, subjects were randomly allocated to one of two groups. The control group received direct SLT intervention three times a week, in addition to daily indirect trained nurse management. The experimental group received indirect management via trained nursing staff responsible for day-to-day management. SLT reviewed subjects fortnightly, unless specifically requested to reassess by nursing staff. Trained nursing staff were defined as any member of the multidisciplinary team who had attended dysphagia screening and management training sessions carried out by SLT. Protocols were devised for both groups and ethical approval for these were gained before commencement of the study.

Outcome measures and results

Twenty subjects were recruited over a five-month period. The median age was eighty-one years (range 70–93). During the course of the study, six subjects died of causes unrelated to dysphagia. Average time since onset of stroke was 3.5 days. Three main outcome measures were used:

1. Length of time taken to achieve a functional swallow (exclusively oral feeding) for a period of seven days with no adverse signs, ie. aspiration, dehydration or malnutrition, as defined by Neumann (1995). Compensatory strategies to reduce the risk of aspiration could be used. These could include head-turning, chin tuck, and double swallow techniques widely used by SLTs to reduce the risk of aspiration by improving airway protection (Logemann, 1983). Diet could be modified in texture, ie. soft but not puree. Fluids could be thickened. This ranged from five to sixty days. The average time for the control group to obtain functional swallow was thirty-two days and for the experimental group twenty-five days.

2. Incidence of chest infection. Within the clinical setting, chest status continues to be used as a measure of functional swallow. As discussed, the link between pneumonia and oropharyngeal dysphagia leading to aspiration of food or liquid has been widely documented (Langmore *et al*, 1998). This proved inconclusive in this study. The only subject who had a diagnosed chest infection was in the control group.

3. Incidence of weight loss. This measure was selected given that dysphagic patients are at risk of malnutrition, decreasing rehabilitation potential and increasing the likelihood of a poor overall outcome. Only six of the twenty subjects had weights taken during the course of the study. Four lost weight and two gained weight.

Discussion

The drive for evidence-based practice produced this piece of work, which took two years from conception to completion. Although statistically insignificant, what knowledge can be gained from the experience?

1. Functional swallow

Functional swallow was the most reliable indicator of patient improvement, but does require close monitoring by well-trained nursing staff to ensure that patients progress through consistencies. The case studies below show specific examples of nurse management. The authors believe that if the nursing staff are well-trained and supported by SLTs, this could form the basis of a larger study.

Bowles (2001) identifies the need for work in partnership across and within professions in order to improve training in this area. Where this takes place, there is no doubt that a full research project could take place. The authors found that responses to nurse questionnaires completed at the end of the study supported Bowles' findings that nurses commonly state pressure of work, fears about competency and low morale to be the main limiting factors to effective screening and — we would also suggest — management of this client group. National competencies for dysphagia, at the time of writing, are about to be piloted in sites across the UK. This should begin to address some of these issues. The project, a joint initiative between the Royal College of Speech and Language Therapists (RCSLT) and the Royal College of Nursing, has been commissioned by the Department of Health (DoH) Care Group Workforce Team. The ultimate aim is to develop the skills, knowledge and ability of SLTs and other healthcare professionals, namely nursing staff, to contribute more effectively to the identification and management of dysphagia.

The authors recommend a combination of broad-based training offered to all those involved in helping stroke patients to eat and drink, where possible incorporating it into induction programmes for new staff and at the level of student nurse training. Further training in screening and management of swallowing problems following a stroke should be offered to all staff working on stroke units, including medical staff. It is suggested locally that most dysphagia screens are carried out by nursing staff and this is reflected in Perry's audit (2001). Hinds and Wiles (1998) state that there are often no clear lines of responsibility for screening and referral to speech and language therapy. Studies have also identified a role for dysphagia link nurses (Heritage, 2003; Davies, 2002) equipping nurses with a wider knowledge-base, a requirement to produce evidence of ward-based patient contact and a remit to initiate the screening and management of dysphagia.

2. Chest status

Chest status was not a reliable outcome measure and the diagnosis of chest infection was problematic. Clinically, SLTs are cautious where there may be a degree of chestiness following oral intake, but not necessarily a diagnosed chest infection. The authors would define chestiness as 'wet or bubbly' chest sounds, which may indicate collection of secretions and/or bolus material in the pharynx, laryngeal vestibule or upper airways. More recent publications have highlighted the complexity of using chest status as an indicator of aspiration of oral intake associated with dysphagia. Perry and Love (2001) state that aspiration is a prerequisite for pneumonia but not all who aspirate develop infection. Normal subjects are known to aspirate without symptoms and little is known about characteristics that may make a person more susceptible to pneumonia, eg. features of aspirate and/or the individual. Langmore (1999) found that poor oral hygiene predisposes patients to chest infection. The literature indicates that higher rates of aspiration pneumonia are found in tube-fed patients (58–67%) than in non-tube-fed patients (14–17%), which is further supported by clinical experience. Documentation in the literature, however, is confusing and contradictory. There is also a suggestion that bedside evaluation of swallow is a poor predictor of aspiration (McCullough et al, 2000). However, within a busy hospital environment, this is the most frequently used method of assessment and is also more appropriate for the older acute stroke patient than videofluoroscopy

(VF). Assessment may usefully be supported with use of cervical auscultation (Zenner, 1995) and pulse oximetry (Smith, 2001). Since the pilot study, there has been a greater use of these assessment tools reported by SLTs to augment bedside evaluation of swallow.

In summary, given the number of variables affecting chest status, a large scale study should consider clear protocols for the following:

- definition of chest infection
- when to use more objective methods of measuring aspiration, such as video fluoroscopy, cervical auscultation and pulse oximetry
- pre-morbid chest status or predisposing factors
- other risk factors such as alternative feeding.

A large enough study with clear protocols for chest status may be the only way to prove one way or another which method of intervention is more successful at reducing rates of chest infection associated with dysphagia.

3. Weight and nutritional status

Weight and nutritional status was, perhaps surprisingly, a difficult measure to use simply because patients were not being weighed. A study by Smithard *et al* (1996) found that nutritional indices, including weight, deteriorated over the first month post-stroke. The *National Service Framework for Older People* (DoH, 2001) recommends attention to nutritional status as good practice. The launch of *The Essence of Care* (2001) resource pack reinforces the need to improve the patient's experience of food and nutrition, and identifies the need to set clear standards for dysphagia. In the light of these recent publications, members of the team should be made more aware of the need for regular weights as best practice. The authors recommend that weighing of subjects is essential within a full study.

Since the present study, there has been research carried out locally on involving carers in the decision-making process regarding appropriate use of alternative feeding methods (Williams, 2003). This is also reflected in the literature (Gordan and Sheehan, 2004).

The way forward

This article has presented to the reader an account of a small-scale pilot project, funded and supported at a local level. The findings have been discussed and, hopefully, will provide an incentive for further study.

Perry and Love (2001), in their systematic review of the literature, ask: 'Can we use the work to improve patient outcomes?' and suggest the question has barely been approached: 'There is work in progress but the potential remains enormous.' This study has provided indications for best practice, but needs to be taken further before we can answer the question: what is the most clinically effective way of managing dysphagia post-stroke?

Case study 1: Maisy

Maisy was seventy-nine years old when she had a stroke. Following screening by nursing staff, she was referred to speech and language therapy for assessment, two days post-stroke. She was assessed by an independent speech and language therapist using research protocol and her swallow was found to be unsafe. It was recommended, in consultation with the multidisciplinary team, that she remain nil by mouth (NBM) and be given alternative feeding.

Maisy was then assigned to the experimental group for nurse management of her dysphagia. She was discharged from the project after thirty-four days when she was managing full oral feeding.

Maisy's progress was reviewed at fourteen days as defined in the research protocol. Research therapists were required to review her medical and nursing care plan only. No verbal prompts were needed. Nursing staff had successfully managed Maisy's spontaneous recovery from NBM status to oral feeding. She had commenced puree diet thirteen days post stroke. At no stage was speech and language therapy advice requested.

Chest status remained clear throughout the study. Maisy's weight was recorded eighteen days and twenty-two days post admission. This was inadequate data for inclusion in the study. On final reassessment by the independent SLT, voice quality, tongue movement, cough to command and reflex cough had improved. However, Maisy continued to have a moderate dysarthria which did require direct SLT intervention.

Case study 2: Bob

Bob was seventy-seven years old. He was referred to speech and language therapy three days post-stroke after dysphagia screening by nursing staff.

Following assessment as in *Case study 1*, he was also assigned to the experimental group. There was in addition evidence of dysphasia and oral dyspraxia, but posture and conscious level were unimpaired. Bob was felt to be at risk of aspirating with thin fluids, but safe on a soft diet — so he was placed on soft diet and thickened fluids.

Seven days into the study, the SLT department was contacted regarding advice for Bob's wife. Fourteen days into the study, when reviewed by research SLT, it was found that he had been placed on a puree diet by nursing staff because they felt that the soft diet was not always reliable and puree was safer. They did, however, observe that he was sometimes coughing on the soft diet. Fourteen days later, when reviewed, Bob was still on a puree diet and thickened fluids. Staff were prompted to screen for thin fluids and to try a soft diet following the guidelines on the dysphagia flowcharts.

Bob was discharged from the project at thirty-five days. Chest status remained clear. Weights were taken on admission and fifteen and twenty-seven days later. There was a weight loss of 1kg. Nursing staff had required prompts and requested support from speech and language therapy. They had, however, shown an awareness of safe swallow by modifying his diet in the early stages.

References

Bowles H (2000) The need for Leadership. *Speech Lang Ther Pract* **Winter edn** 2000

British Dietetic Association (2002) National Descriptors for Texture Modification. Royal College of Speech and Language Therapists, London

CODA Collaboration Dysphagia Audit (1997) Guidelines for Screening and Management of Stroke Patients with Dysphagia. http://ncl.ac.uk/stroke-research-unit/coda/coguide.htm

Dangerfield L, Sullivan R (1999) Screening and managing dysphagia after stroke. *Nurs Times* **95**(19): 44–5

Davalos A (1996) Effect of malnutrition after acute stroke on clinical outcome. *Stroke* **27**: 1028–32

Davies S (2002) Interdisciplinary approach to the management of dysphagia. *Prof Nurse* **18**(1): 22–5

DePippo KL, Holas MA, Reding MJ (1992) Validation of the 3oz water swallow test for aspiration following stroke. *Arch Neurol* **49**: 1259–61

DePippo KL, Holas MA, Reding MJ (1994) The Burke Screening Test for Dysphagia: validation of its use in patients with stroke. *Arch Phys Med Rehab* **75**(12): 1284–6

Ellul J, Barer D, Fall S (1997) Improving detection and management of swallowing problems in acute stroke: a multidisciplinary centre study. *Cerebrovasc Dis* **6**(suppl 2): 152–3

DoH (2001) Exploring the role and contribution of the nurse in the multi-professional rehabilitation team. *Essence of Care Resource Pack*. ENB.

DoH (2001) *National Service Framework for Older People*. DoH, London

Gariballa S (1998) Nutritional status of hospitalised acute stroke patients. *Br J Nutr* **79**: 481–7

Gordon C, Hewer R, Wade D (1987) Dysphagia in acute stroke. *BMJ* **295**: 411–14

Gordon M, Sheena K (2004) Artificial intelligence: making decisions about artificial nutrition and hydration. *J Nutr Health Aging* **8**(4): 254–6

Hamdy *et al* (1998) Recovery of swallowing after dysphagic stroke relates to functional reorganization in the intact motor cortex. *Gastroenterology* **115**: 1104–12

Heritage M (2003) Swallowing caseloads. *RCSLT Bulletin* **April**: 10–11

Hinds NP, Wiles CM (1998) Assessment of swallowing and referral to speech and language therapists in acute stroke. *Q J Med* **91**: 829–35

Langmore S (1998) Predictors of aspiration: how important is dysphagia? *Dysphagia* **13**: 69–81

Logemann J (1983) *Evaluation and Treatment of Swallowing Disorders*. Pro Ed, Austin (Texas)

McCullough G, Wertz R, Rosenbek J, Mills R, Ross K, Ashford J (2000) Inter- and intra-judge reliability of a clinical examination of swallowing in adults. *Dysphagia* **15**: 58–67

Neumann S, Bartolome G, Buchhotz M, Proseigel M (1995) Swallowing therapy of neurologic patients: correlation of outcome with pre-treatment variables and therapeutic methods. *Dysphagia* **10**: 1–5

Nilsson H, Ekberg O *et al* (1996) Quantative aspects of swallowing in an elderly non-dysphagic population. *Dysphagia* **11**: 180–4

Patteson (1996) Dysphagia in the elderly. *Family Physicians (Can)* **42**: 925–32

Perry L, Love C (2001) Screening for dysphagia and aspiration in acute stroke. *Dysphagia* **16**: 7–18

Royal College of Physicians (2004) *Clinical Guidelines for Stroke. 2nd edn.* Royal College of Physicians, London

Royal College of Speech and Language Therapy (2004) *Clinical Guidelines for Dysphagia.* RCSLT, London

Smith H, Lee S *et al* (2000) The combination of bedside swallowing assessment and oxygen saturation monitoring of swallowing in acute stroke: a safe and humane screening tool. *Age Ageing* **29**: 495–9

Smithard DG, O'Neill P *et al* (1996) Complications and outcome after acute stroke: does dysphagia matter? *Stroke* **27**(7): 1200–04

Smithard D, O'Neill P, England R *et al* (1997) The natural history of dysphagia following stroke. *Dysphagia* **12**: 188–93

Travers P (1999) Post stroke dysphagia: implications for nurses. *Rehabil Nurs* **24**(2): 69–73

Zenner P (1995) Using cervical auscultation in the clinical dysphagia examination in long term care. *Dysphagia* **10**: 27–31

CHAPTER 12

Enabling people with aphasia to discuss quality of life

Joan Murphy

This chapter describes a study that examined the effectiveness of Talking Mats, a low-tech communication framework, in allowing people with communication difficulties as a result of stroke to discuss their quality of life. The study included twelve people in different residential situations. The findings have implications for consumer involvement in rehabilitation.

Stroke can have many sudden and devastating consequences on a person's lifestyle. Changes include problems with mobility, activities of daily living (ADL), communication and relationships. Damaged communication is one of the most distressing aspects (Holland, 1998). Yet, the period immediately after a stroke is often the time when crucial decisions affecting the person's future have to be made and failure to communicate can be distressing for patients, relatives and staff.

In Scotland, guidelines are available on the management of patients with stroke during the acute medical phase (Scottish Intercollegiate Guidelines Network [SIGN], 1997), but details on how people with stroke will be consulted are missing. It is not clear how people will be involved in making informed choices about their future (and much changed) life, or when decisions are being made before discharged from hospital. Although SIGN Guideline 24, which discusses rehabilitation and discharge planning, recognises the importance of aims and objectives being established and agreed by all parties, there is no acknowledgement of the difficulties a person with aphasia will have in understanding and/or expressing his/her views on rehabilitation issues. SIGN Guideline 24 states that:

> *Information should be presented both verbally and in written form to the patient and family or carers.*

However, once the person returns to the community, there are no clear guidelines and many more variable factors that determine the person's quality of life.

Quality of life measures

Having examined the tools that are currently available for measuring quality of life, there appear to be no measures that satisfactorily allow people with communication difficulties to express their point of view. Many existing measures are based on medical rather then social criteria, eg. the Nottingham Health Profile (Hunt, 1984), and focus on the negative aspects of quality of life, such as pain, lack of sleep and social isolation, eg. the Hospital and Anxiety and Depression Scales (HADS) (Zigmond and Snaith, 1983).

Although some measures attempt to include the person's perceptions, such as the 'Short Form 36' (Ware *et al*, 1993), they do not consider the difficulties with speech, language, fatigue, poor hand control and literacy that a person may have while completing the measure. The book *Measuring Health* (Bowling, 1998) describes a wide range of health measures, but none of them consider the specific difficulties people with severe communication difficulties have in completing these measures.

A search of the literature revealed little concerning quality of life measures for people with aphasia. Hinckley (1998) sent a questionnaire to 145 adults with aphasia, asking them to provide a self-rating on life-satisfaction. She suggested that the respondents' difficulty in completing a linguistically loaded, multiple-page questionnaire resulted in a low response rate (21%). Holland (1998) reviewed different approaches to functional outcome measures, including those that claim to be specifically designed for people with aphasia. However, none of these approaches addressed the problems of administering a test to those who have difficulty in understanding and/ or expressing themselves. She states that 'no currently available measure examines the effect of communication problems on the quality of life post-stroke'.

Moreover, discussions with a number of speech and language therapists working in departments with stroke patients in Scotland revealed that none were aware of any suitable quality of life measures being used for stroke patients either with or without communication difficulties.

There is therefore a pressing need to develop a tool that will allow people with a communication difficulty to be included in discussion and decisions about their lives. As part of a previous research project, Talking Mats (Murphy, 1998a, 1998b) was developed, which enabled people with cerebral palsy and communication difficulties to express their thoughts and views. A research project was then undertaken on the use of Talking Mats with people with motor neurone disease to discuss their quality of life (Murphy, 1999). The study described in this chapter examined whether or not Talking Mats could be used successfully with people with aphasia. The project was funded by the Chief Scientist Office of the Scottish Executive and was completed in February 2000. Ethical permission was obtained from the ethics committee for the Forth Valley Health Board.

Method

The framework is based on three sets of picture symbols that are presented to the person with a communication difficulty. The following areas were covered:

1. Issues that are relevant for quality of life
2. Factors relating to each quality of life issue
3. Emotions — in order to allow participants to indicate their general feeling about each factor.

The main issues presented were people, home, health, work, indoor and outdoor interests. For those participants on the acute and long-stay wards, home was replaced by ward. A variety of different factors were displayed for each issue. The factors were selected following discussion with speech and language therapists (SLTs), ward staff and the participants. The range of emotions — happy, content, not sure, worried, angry — was altered depending on the receptive abilities of the participant, eg. for some people the number was reduced from five to three.

Each 'mat' has a range of emotion symbols along the top (*Figure 12.1*) and focuses on a single issue. The relevant factors are presented to each participant, who then selects the ones that are important to him/her and places them under the appropriate emotion, thus building up a composite picture of his/her views. Picture Communication Symbols (PCS) produced on the software package Boardmaker™ were used.

The Talking Mats have a number of distinctive features, which are crucial for people with communication difficulties when considering quality of life issues. This framework ensured that:

- It is simple and enjoyable to use.
- It is non-threatening in that there are no right or wrong answers.
- It does not require literacy.
- The pictorial symbols are cognitively easy to access without appearing childish.
- The strands of the issues to be discussed are separated into manageable chunks, which assists comprehension.
- The factors that influence the quality of life issues can be easily personalised for each individual.
- The pictorial symbols can be used to augment the participant's existing communication system or used as an alternative to speech.
- People with limited hand control and/or those who become easily fatigued can use the Talking Mats by eye-pointing or using listener scanning.
- The participants can take as long as they need to consider, select and move the pictures around. They can also change them until they are satisfied that the final composite picture truly represents what they mean.
- The final pictorial representation can be photographed as a permanent record of the participant's views, and used to bring about change.
- The results can be compared by carrying out the interview on different occasions with the same person.

Participants

Twelve people living in four different residential situations — at home, with family, home alone, acute ward awaiting discharge, or in a long-stay hospital ward — took part in the project. The twelve participants had varying degrees of aphasia: five had both severe receptive and expressive aphasia; three had moderate receptive and expressive aphasia; three had mild receptive and expressive aphasia; and one was predominantly dysarthric.

The participants were interviewed using the Talking Mats framework. The interviews were video-recorded and subsequently analysed using cognitive mapping (Jones, 1985). In cognitive mapping, the factors relating to specific issues are extrapolated, and a map is drawn to represent each participant's views and the connections between them. Individual maps are then combined into more complex maps that group participants' views to compare patterns and highlight unique reflections. Digital photographs were taken of the completed mats.

Results

All twelve people were able to express their views using the symbols. From participants' comments and from observations of their non-verbal communication, the completion of the mats appeared to be a meaningful and satisfying activity. It provided an opportunity for the most able participants to consider their current lifestyle and possible future changes. For some, it offered a chance to express their thoughts to their spouses — something that they had not done before. Others were able to indicate satisfaction or dissatisfaction with their residential situation. The following short summaries illustrate some of the views that people were able to express.

At home with family

Those who lived at home with their families rated family members' contributions to their quality of life highly. This was demonstrated by the participants placing the pictures representing close family members at the most positive end of the range of emotions. They were also able to express the ways in which different family members affected their lives. For example, one man indicated that one of his daughters improved his quality of life more than the other (who had two young, boisterous children, who made him feel exhausted).

Spouses were present during the interview with three participants who lived with their families. All were surprised by some of the views expressed by the participants. In one example, the participant indicated that he disliked going out in the fresh air, whereas his wife had assumed that he enjoyed being taken outside in his wheelchair *(Figure 12.1)*.

At home alone

All three participants who lived alone indicated that the garden was a source of anxiety as they were no longer able to look after it. Two people indicated that some family members upset them and two found shopping stressful. The following example shows how swimming, shopping and the garden frustrated the man who completed this mat *(Figure 12.2)*. He also requested a second car symbol to express how his car hampered his life when it was off the road, but greatly improved his quality of life when it was working.

Acute ward

The main observation from this group was that the Talking Mats provided a trigger for the participants to describe their lives and interests. It could also serve as a framework for planning discharge, as it highlighted what people regarded as important in their lives. For example, the man who completed the mat shown in *Figure 12.3* was easy-going about most factors, but was clear that having enough space and his own privacy were very important to him.

Long stay

All three participants in long-stay wards were unhappy with the quality of service they received, which in turn affected their quality of life. The main areas of discontent were lack of privacy and lack of involvement in decision making, as shown in *Figure 12.4*.

Ethical issues

Talking Mats allowed some people to raise issues of frustration and unhappiness with their situation. Ten participants indicated frustration with aspects of their quality of life, in particular, speech and mobility difficulties. Three people living in long-stay wards expressed unhappiness with their residential situation. During the interviews, care was taken to acknowledge the participants' feelings and to restore and affirm their feelings of self-worth. For example, one participant initially indicated that she felt that there were no people in her life who were important to her. However, the researcher was able to use her completed mat to show her that she had selected a number of people who she considered improved her quality of life *(Figure 12.5)*.

The completed mats provided evidence that life was not as negative as some people had first thought, while for others it highlighted areas that could be altered to improve their quality of life. For example, one man indicated that he felt upset that he could no longer read, and as a result his carer took him to the library and borrowed some audio books for him *(Figure 12.6)*. His key worker also investigated the possibility of getting him involved with the local photography club.

Effects of aphasia

Patterns of language difficulty only affected the ability of the participants to use the framework in that people with a receptive difficulty took longer to complete the interview. However, they found it just as fulfilling (in some cases more so) as those whose speech was only mildly affected. It is significant to acknowledge the factors that people omitted, as well as the factors they selected as being important in their lives. For example, all but two participants omitted their medical consultant as an important factor.

Feedback

The author believes that giving feedback is an essential part of research and that the research process should provide direct benefits to the study participants. With the exception of one (who had become very ill), all participants were visited a few weeks after their interview and were given photographs of their completed 'mats'. It was stressed that it was their choice if they wanted to show their 'mats' to anyone else. Most of them indicated that they wanted to show them to their SLTs.

At the feedback visit, all participants affirmed that their involvement in the research had been both enjoyable and interesting. No-one indicated that they had found it distressing or negative. They all believed that the issues presented to them had covered the main aspects of their lives. Spouses were present with the three participants who lived with their families, and all took on board the views of their husbands, even though they were not what they expected. For example, one spouse had not realised that her husband missed his dog, but subsequently got another one from the RSPCA. Using photographs in conjunction with Talking Mats allows feedback to be given, not only to the participants but also (with their permission) to the family, carers and professionals. For several participants, some aspects of their lives changed in a positive way as a result of the study.

Conclusion

Although this was a small study, it indicated that the Talking Mats framework has the potential to help people with a communication difficulty as a result of stroke express their views about quality of life issues. It helped participants to identify the factors that were important to them and indicate how these either improved or hampered their lives. Using this interactive and visual format appears to be a more comfortable and successful method of generating information for people with a communication difficulty than a structured interview or questionnaire. People were allowed to take as long as they required to consider, select and move the pictures around. They could also change them until they were happy that the final composite picture truly represented what they meant.

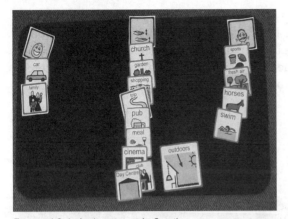

Figure 12.1: At home with family.

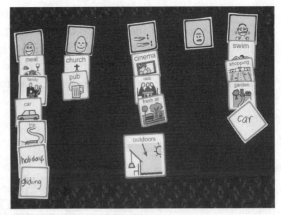

Figure 12.2: At home alone.

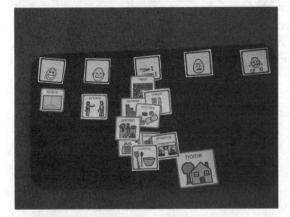

Figure 12.3: Acute ward.

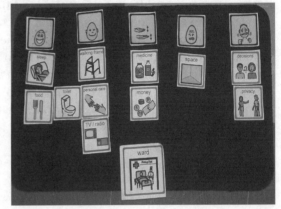

Figure 12.4: Long stay.

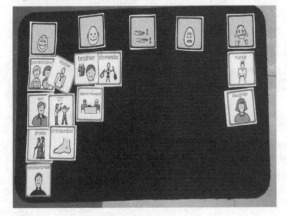

Figure 12.5: People.

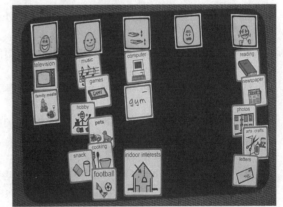

Figure 12.6: Indoor interests.

However, it must be acknowledged that it also raised issues that were painful for some people. For example, eight of the ten who completed the health mat indicated their frustration with their communication difficulty. Another limitation was the difficulty for someone with a severe aphasia to express unexpected ideas not previously considered by the researcher, though several succeeded by using gestures, eg. one man used a gesture to indicate his concern about a cardiac problem.

Future initiatives

The method needs to be refined so that it can be used with a larger sample of people in order to show reliability and validity. If reliable, it will produce the same results when applied to the same participants at different times and by different interviewers when there is no evidence of change. However, it should also show that it is sensitive to change. Validity will be shown by the degree of confidence that can be placed on the inferences drawn from the mats. The author is currently involved in using the Talking Mats to adapt a discharge questionnaire used in an acute stroke rehabilitation unit to include people with aphasia. She is also involved in a research project looking at the use of Talking Mats with frail older people in nursing homes. Ways of providing training in the use of Talking Mats for other staff involved in health, social work, education and housing are currently being examined.

Implications

Some of the possible implications of Talking Mats for people with a stroke are:

- They can be used as a stimulus to consider quality of life in a positive and affirming way.
- They can be used as an initial screening to obtain an overall picture of the participant's views, both in hospital and at home, and provide an opportunity to return and explore issues in more detail.
- They can be used to consult people before discharge from hospital and provide information to ward staff and social work staff.
- They can be used to allow people to comment on the quality of service, such as food, privacy, warmth and staff attitudes in hospitals and nursing homes.
- They can inform family/carers of the views expressed in a tangible way.

The real value of the tool, however, will depend on how a person's quality of life is improved by family, carers, staff and patients, and the changes made as a result of the views expressed on the Talking Mats.

Talking Mats is the copyright of University of Stirling and is available from the AAC Research Unit, University of Stirling. The Picture Communication Symbols (PCS) are copyright ©1981–1999 Mayer Johnson Co., and are used with kind permission from Mayer-Johnson Co., PO Box 1579, Solana Beach, CA 92075, USA

References

Bowling A (1998) *Measuring Health: a Review of Quality of Life Measurement Scales.* Open University Press, Buckinghamshire

Hinckley JJ (1998) Predictors of lifestyle satisfaction among younger adults with chronic aphasia. *Aphasiology* **12**(7/8): 509–18

Holland AL (1998) Functional outcome assessment of aphasia following left hemisphere stroke. *Semin Speech Language* **19**(3): 249–59

Hunt SM (1984) Nottingham Health Profile. In: Wenger NK, Mattson ME, Furberg CD *et al* (eds) *Assessment of Quality of Life in Clinical Trials of Cardiovascular Therapies.* Le Jacq, New York

Jones S (1985) The analysis of depth interviews. In: Walker R (ed) *Applied Qualitative Research.* Gower Publishing Company Ltd, Aldershot: 56–70

Murphy J (1998a) Talking Mats. *Speech Language Ther Pract* **Autumn:** 11–14

Murphy J (1998b) Helping people with severe communication difficulties to express their views: a low-tech tool. *Commun Matters* **12**(2): 9–11

Murphy J (1999) Enabling people with motor neurone disease to discuss their quality of life. *Commun Matters* **13**(2): 2–6

Scottish Intercollegiate Guidelines Network (1997) *Management of Patients with Stroke (Guideline Nos. 13, 14, 20 and 24).* Scottish Intercollegiate Guidelines Network, Edinburgh

Ware JE, Snow KK, Kosinski M, Gandek B (1993) *SF-36 Health Survey: Manual and Interpretation Guide.* The Health Institute, New England Medical Centre, Boston, Massachusetts

Zigmond AS, Snaith RP (1983) The Hospital and Anxiety Depression Scale. *Acta Psychiatr Scand* **67:** 361–70

CHAPTER 13

Care of residents with post-stroke communication problems

Terri Horton

Imagine that you are enjoying yourself in a familiar place with familiar people but cannot understand what they are saying. You try to speak, but all you produce is a garbled noise. How would you feel? Frustrated, frightened or confused?

Life-shattering change

This kind of situation has been experienced by many people who had communication problems after a stroke. It is a sudden and devastating change.

Bryan and Drew (1989) found that just over half of all residents in residential care settings had some communication difficulties. Many of these difficulties were the result of a stroke. The ability of care staff to recognise such problems and to act in ways that promote good communication is essential to enhance the quality of life of residents with post-stroke communication problems.

Why do we communicate?

It seems to be a simple question, but it is worth taking a little time to consider all the situations in which communication is used. Some of them are shown in *Table 13.1*. Problems with communication affect many of these situations, and language then often becomes restricted to answering questions that others ask (Parr *et al*, 1997). Obviously, it is a very frustrating situation not to be able to join in a conversation, tell a joke, or even just say, 'Hello, how are you?' to a fellow resident.

Providers of care must make sure that they do not limit how residents interact with people and thereby deny them the opportunity to use their language in as rich a way as possible.

Problems of communication

Communication problems are most common after a stroke that affects the left side of the brain. This is because, for most people, the left hemisphere of the brain is dominant for language. For a small number of left-handed people, however, the right hemisphere is dominant and language problems can occur after a stroke affecting this side of the brain (Beaumont, 1974).

There are a number of problems that can affect communication. The most common of them are aphasia, dysarthria and dyspraxia. This article looks at each of these in turn, and then describes ways of removing the barriers that frustrate people who may have these difficulties.

The way society views health and health care has moved away from a medical model towards an approach based on a social model. This is also the case for the way in which people with communication problems are treated. The barriers to effective communication and the question of how we can remove them are now the most important issues, and carers are more than ever concerned with what can be done to enable communication to take place rather than just to focus on the problems themselves (Jordan and Kaiser, 1996).

Table 13.1: Functions of communication
❖ Greeting
❖ Expressing emotion
❖ Asking for things or information
❖ Commenting and giving opinions
❖ Humour and telling jokes
❖ Getting our own way or arguing
❖ Thinking and problem-solving
❖ Making friends
❖ Imagining or daydreaming
❖ Giving information

Aphasia

In England, the terms 'aphasia' and 'dysphasia' are used interchangeably. In this article, the term 'aphasia' will be used. Aphasia is a difficulty with language, and people with this condition can have problems with any or all of the following:

* talking
* understanding what other people say
* reading and writing
* understanding and using numbers.

It is vital to emphasise, however, that people with aphasia are able to think clearly, know what they feel, and can make their own decisions — so they should be treated as competent adults. As Kagan (1995) has shown, even those with severe communication problems can demonstrate their competence and participate in decision-making. All too often, people with aphasia have described situations in which they were ignored or treated as though they were no longer intelligent people (Edelman and Greenwood, 1992; Parr *et al*, 1997).

The difficulties that arise in aphasia can be mild, moderate or severe. People with mild problems

Table 13.2: Muscles used for speaking

❖ Muscles of the chest used for breathing

❖ Muscles of the larynx (voice box) to produce voice

❖ Muscles of the face, lips, tongue and throat

may be able to follow what is being said but have difficulty in larger groups when conversation is quicker and speakers change rapidly. They may be able to say or write down what they would like to express with only occasional problems in finding the right word or spelling. Someone with severe problems may be unable to recognise simple words or gestures, or to produce meaningful words, or they may get stuck on the same word or sound whenever they speak (perseveration).

It is important to remember that however severe the communication problem may be, residents with communication problems are still competent adults with the ability to think and feel, and they should be treated with respect and involved in decisions about their care.

Dysarthria

This is a result of the stroke damaging the workings of the muscles involved in speaking (*Table 13.2*). The muscles may have been weakened or become stiff and poorly coordinated. Speech can therefore sound slurred or harsh and be difficult to understand. The volume may be uncontrolled and the rhythm jerky. Dysarthria may be made worse by poorly fitting dentures, so it is important to check that they fit well.

If the dysarthria occurs on its own, the person with this condition will not have the difficulties with word-finding or understanding associated with aphasia. However, sometimes dysarthria and aphasia can occur together.

Dyspraxia

Dyspraxia affects the conscious coordination of the movements needed to produce speech and is not caused by paralysis or any muscular problems. A person may struggle to produce a sound or be unable to sequence the sounds that make up a word.

This is a very frustrating condition and one that is difficult to appreciate. For example, some clients may be completely unable to put out their tongue when you ask them to, but can automatically put out their tongue to lick their lips, for example, if eating a sugary doughnut. It is the 'automatic' nature of the second activity that allows the movement to occur easily.

Removing the barriers to communication

To help someone understand information:

- Speak more slowly than usual (while remembering that the person you are speaking to is an adult).
- Write messages down by using the important (key) words.
- Use simple diagrams or illustrations.
- Use simple gestures to accompany speech.
- Do not shout or speak too loudly.
- Recap to make sure that the resident has understood.
- Allow plenty of time for the message to be understood.

To help people with communication problems get their message across:

- Allow plenty of time for him or her to speak.
- Listen carefully and do not interrupt.
- Try to reduce any background noise or distractions.
- Pay attention to the tone of the voice and facial expression, as these can give useful clues.
- Do not finish the words or sentences for the person with the communication difficulty.
- Encourage that person to use drawing, writing or gesture, if possible.
- Encourage the person to use any communication aids, such as a word list, picture book or personal portfolio.
- Be honest if all of what someone has said is not understood.
- Encourage the person with the communication difficulty to indicate yes or no.
- Check back to ensure that all has been understood.

Other issues

- Visual problems, such as field defects, double vision and recognition problems, can have an impact on someone's ability to communicate. Making sure that patients wear their glasses is also important, as they may not see people or writing clearly.
- A lot of effort is needed for concentrating, thinking, listening and talking. It is important to try to find the time of day when the person is most alert and also to encourage frequent rests.
- Communication problems can vary from day to day and be worse if the person is tired, upset or anxious.
- Sometimes people can swear even when they cannot say very much else. They may be unaware of doing it, and it may be something they did not previously do. This can be upsetting both for themselves, their family and for care staff, and it is important to understand that this is often the result of the stroke. The swear words may be the only 'automatic' words that come out when the person is trying to express emotion. It usually does improve over time.
- It may happen that people who have spoken English for most of their lives, but whose first language is not English, may revert to their first language after a stroke. It is thought that if two languages are learned at different times, they are stored in different parts of the brain,

and so the stroke may have damaged one area while leaving the first language intact. It is important to have an interpreter to help people with this kind of problem communicate.

- The brain's ability to control weeping and laughing may be affected by a stroke, and some stroke patients may cry and laugh for no reason or can start to cry at a kind word or a sad scene on television. This does improve over time, but it is helpful if the carer stays calm, avoids joining in with the laughter, tries to change the subject, and gives the person time to regain control.

- Positioning may be important. Communication usually happens between people who are facing each other at the same height. If people are positioned at different heights (eg. one is standing while the other is sitting), stand too close or too far apart from each other, or sit in chairs that are arranged in such a way that comfortable and direct communication is difficult, the impression that one of the speakers is not interested or does not consider the other speaker important may be created. Carers should be at the same height, in good light and facing residents when talking.

- As with other 'automatic' modes of speech, such as saying the alphabet and days of the week, the words to songs are often retained after a stroke. It is often the case that when a familiar tune is heard (Christmas carols, hymns or popular songs), the person who has suffered from a stroke can sing the words quite accurately. Unfortunately, this does not mean that speech is returning quickly, but it can give someone enjoyment to sing along to well-known tunes.

Recovery

It is difficult to estimate how long recovery may take, particularly soon after a stroke. In the first few days, the brain attempts to repair and recover damaged functions.

Recovery takes time and people may not recover their communication skills as quickly as other skills. People with aphasia may never be able to communicate in the same way as they did before the stroke. Aphasia can, however, continue to improve, and many people see progress a long time after their stroke.

Speech and language therapy

A person with communication problems after a stroke should see a speech and language therapist (SLT). The SLT will assess the problem and help find the easiest ways for the person to communicate. The therapist will also know of other services in the area that can provide ongoing support to the person with the communication problems and their family (such as the Stroke Association and Speakability). If someone has not seen an SLT, they should be referred, and this can be done directly or via a GP. If someone has attended therapy or is still doing so, it is useful to contact the SLT to find out what things can be done to help the person. Activities and exercises can help build up relationships and to give the person confidence in communicating.

As aphasia is something that a person lives with, any therapy must reflect the environment and interests of that person to have any relevance. Pound *et al* (2000) give some examples of this in their book. There are other resources as well, including training packages and information for carers and people with communication problems. The most accessible include those produced by the Stroke Association and Speakability and, most notably, The Aphasia Handbook (Parr *et al*, 1999). The challenge for us all is to make our approach to communication one that breaks down the barriers and enables people to participate fully in all aspects of their lives.

References

Beaumont J (1974) Handedness and hemisphere function. In: Dimond S, Beaumont J (eds) *Hemisphere Function in the Human Brain*. Elek, London

Bryan KL, Drew S (1989) A survey of communication disability in an elderly population in residential care. *Int J Rehabil Res* **12**(3): 330–3

Edelman G, Greenwood R (eds) (1992) *Jumbly Words and Rights Where Wrongs Should Be: the Experience of Aphasia from the Inside*. Far Communications, Kibworth

Jordan L, Kaiser W (1996) *Aphasia — a Social Approach*. Chapman & Hall, London

Kagan A (1995) Revealing the competence of aphasic adults through conversation: a challenge to health professionals. *Top Stroke Rehabil* **2**(1): 15–28

Parr S, Byng S, Gilpin S (1997) *Talking About Aphasia: Living With Loss of Language After Stroke*. Open University Press, Milton Keynes

Parr S, Pound C, Byng S, Long B (1999) *The Aphasia Handbook*. Connect Press, London

Pound C, Parr S, Lindsay J, Woolf C (2000) *Beyond Aphasia — Therapies for Living with Communication Disability*. Winslow, Oxford

Useful websites

The Royal College of Speech and Language Therapists (RCSLT) — www.rcslt.org

Speakability — www.speakability.org.uk

The Stroke Association — www.stroke.org.uk

Evaluating current practice in the provision of written information to stroke patients and their carers

Tammy Hoffman, Kryss McKenna, Linda Worrall, Stephen J Read

The study described in this chapter aimed to determine current practice in the provision of written information to fifty-seven stroke patients and their carers. It also explored their informational needs while in hospital and six months later and examined the suitability of the written materials received, comparing readability levels to participants' general reading ability. While in hospital, 22.8% of patients and 41.7% of carers received written information, yet 91.2% of patients and 100% of carers wanted information. More than half of the participants wanted information on preventing strokes, causes and risk factors of stroke, recovery, what a stroke is, stroke-related medications and sources of further information. At six months after stroke, 75.5% of patients and all carers wanted further information. The mean SMOG readability level of the written materials received was equivalent to a grade 11 level of education, compared with the patients' mean reading ability, which was equivalent to a 7th–8th grade reading level. The authors conclude that stroke patients and their carers want substantially more information than they are receiving, both while in hospital and six months later. The majority of written information that is distributed to these people is unsuitable in terms of readability levels and other factors.

Hoffman T, McKenna K, Worrall L, Read SJ (2004) Evaluating current practice in the provision of written information to stroke patients and their carers. Int J Ther Rehabil *11(7): 303–10*

The education of stroke patients and their carers should be an integral component of stroke management. Patient education can allay anxiety, enhance compliance and adjustment, and increase satisfaction (O'Mahoney *et al*, 1997). In chronic diseases such as stroke, education gives patients the skills to self-manage their disease, which can reduce disease burden and improve quality of life (Cooper *et al*, 2001). Because stroke recovery can be enhanced by the involvement of family members, they should also routinely receive education (Evans *et al*, 1988). Written information offers message consistency, can be referred to when required, and aids recall (Bernier, 1993). While patients generally want written information (Webber, 1990), few receive it about stroke (Wellwood *et al*, 1994; Hanger *et al*, 1998).

Educational materials are only effective if they provide information that patients and their families want. While most health professionals think they know what patients need to know (Doak *et al*, 2001), in previous work, 75% of patients and 79% of carers reported that their informational needs were not completely met while in hospital (Eames *et al*, 2003). The informational needs of stroke patients and their carers change over time (van Veenendaal *et al*, 1996; Wiles *et al*, 1998). Consequently, patients' and carers' informational needs should be established at critical points, such as before discharge and at post-discharge intervals, to ensure that information exchange is individualised.

For patient education to improve knowledge and health behaviour, patients must understand the information that is provided. The comprehensibility of written materials is influenced by the material's readability and the patient's reading ability. Readability refers to the degree of difficulty involved in reading and understanding written text (Jimenez, 1994). Other factors, such as lay-out, graphics, literacy demand and cultural appropriateness, also affect the suitability of written health education materials (Doak *et al*, 2001).

While research about the readability and suitability of written stroke education materials is limited, previous studies have concluded that educational materials are often written at a reading level too high for patients (Estrada *et al*, 2000; Sullivan and O'Conor, 2001). Although a number of studies have examined the informational needs of stroke patients and their carers (Wellwood *et al*, 1994; van Veenendaal *et al*, 1996; Hanger *et al*, 1998; Wiles *et al*, 1998), none has examined the readability and suitability of the written materials received or the reading ability of patients and carers. The aims of the study described in this chapter were to:

- Determine current practice in providing stroke patients and carers with written information, including the proportion who receive it, their satisfaction with it, and its content and source.
- Examine the informational needs of stroke patients and carers while in hospital and six months later.
- Evaluate the readability levels and suitability of written materials that patients and carers receive and compare readability levels to stroke patients' and carers' general reading ability.

Method

Participants

Participants were patients who had been admitted to the stroke unit of a major metropolitan public hospital between February and July, 2002. Informal carers were invited to participate if they were present at the patient's interview. Eligibility criteria were that the participants:

- Had had a stroke or were the informal carer of a person who had had a stroke.
- Lived within 50 km of the hospital.
- Had a reported English proficiency level, corrected hearing and vision and communication status adequate to participate in an interview and complete assessment tasks.
- Did not have a reported or observable dementia.

For patients with aphasia, the stroke unit speech pathologist helped the interviewer in determining their suitability for an interview.

Hospital interviews

Eligible patients were invited to participate in the study up to two days before their discharge. Clinical information (type of stroke, side of stroke, stroke-related impairments and number of previous strokes) was obtained from the medical records. A face-to-face semi-structured interview was held with participants and a questionnaire developed for this study was administered. The questions were informed from previous research (Eames *et al*, 2003) and a literature review. All interviews were completed by the first author. Ethical clearance to conduct this study was obtained from university and hospital committees.

Participants provided sociodemographic details, including date of birth, living situation before stroke (ie. alone, with partner, with family, with friend or other) and years of formal education completed (*Table 14.1*).

Participants were asked if they had received any written information about stroke while they (if the patient) or their family member or friend (if the carer) had been in hospital. If they reported receiving written information, they were asked to provide details about what they had received, who received it (patient, carer or both), its source, if they had read it and if not, why not. If read, participants' satisfaction with the content and presentation of each written material was assessed on a 10-point vertical visual analogue scale (with 1=not satisfied and 10=extremely satisfied). Participants were asked to identify the positive and negative features of the material/s received.

To determine informational needs, participants were asked:

1. If they had any unanswered questions about stroke.
2. To identify from a list of twenty-four stroke-related topics (generated from earlier pilot studies) which topics they would have liked information about and their preferred format for receiving that information.

Finally, participants' reading ability was assessed using the Rapid Estimate of Adult Literacy in Medicine (REALM) (Murphy *et al*, 1993). This assessment requires sixty-six medical terms to be read and pronounced, with raw scores converted into grade estimates.

The written materials received were examined for readability using the SMOG readability formula (McLaughlin, 1969) and for suitability using the Suitability Assessment of Materials checklist (Doak *et al*, 1996b). In the SMOG, thirty sentences are selected, ten each from the beginning, middle and end, and words of three or more syllables are counted. Grade levels are then obtained by using the SMOG conversion table. The Suitability Assessment of Materials checklist consists of twenty-two items grouped under six factors, namely:

- content
- literacy demand
- graphics
- layout or typography
- learning stimulation or motivation
- cultural appropriateness.

Table 14.1: Sociodemographic and clinical characteristics of participants

Sociodemographic and clinical characteristics		Patients (n=57)	Carers	
			Hospital (n=12)	Follow-up (n=9)
Mean age (standard deviation; range)		72.21 years (13.39; 35–92)	61.27 years (11.44; 42–83)	69.9 years (9.4; 50–81)
Sex	Male	52.6%	25%	33%
	Female	47.4%	75%	77%
Type of stroke (no. patients; percentage):	TACI	4 (7.0)		
	PACI	15 (26.3)		
	POCI	5 (8.8)		
	LACI	28 (49.1)		
	ICH	3 (5.3)		
	TIA	2 (3.5)	Not applicable	
Side of stroke (no. patients; percentage):	Right	23 (40.4)		
	Left	34 (59.6)		
No. patients with first stroke (percentage)		44 (77.2)		
No. patients with aphasia (percentage)		15 (26.3)		
Mean no. years of formal education completed (standard deviation; range)		9.2 (2.9; 2–18)	9.0 (1.9; 6–12)	8.7 (1.9; 7–12)
Relationship of carer to patient (no. patients; percentage):	Spouse/partner		7 (58.3)	9 (100.0)
	Daughter		2 (16.7)	
	Son-in-law	Not applicable	1 (8.3)	
	Mother		2 (16.7)	

TACI=total anterior circulation infarct; PACI=partial anterior circulation infarct; POCI=posterior circulation infarct; LACI=lacunar infarct; ICH=intracerebral haemorrhage; TIA=transient ischaemic attack

Items are rated in terms of the degree to which they meet set criteria, on a scale of 2, 1, 0 or 'not applicable'. Total scores are converted into percentages (percentage=total score/possible total score for that written material) and are interpreted using the following guide: 70–100%=superior material; 40–69%=adequate material; 0–39%=unsuitable material.

Follow-up interviews

Participants were contacted six months after the hospital interview for a follow-up interview, which was conducted in participants' homes. Participants were asked the same questions they had been asked in the initial interview, except they were asked if they had received any written information about stroke since the previous interview.

Results

Sociodemographic and clinical characteristics

Hospital interviews were completed for fifty-seven patients and twelve carers. Sociodemographic characteristics of participants, as well as patients' clinical characteristics, are shown in *Table 14.1*.

Follow-up interviews were conducted with forty-nine patients and nine carers. Of the eight patients not followed up, two were deceased and six could not be contacted. Nine carers interviewed in hospital could not be contacted for interview. Six carers interviewed at follow-up had not been interviewed in hospital. Demographics for the follow-up carer sample are included in *Table 14.1*. The mean time from stroke onset to the follow-up interview was 186 days (standard deviation=12, range=164–219).

Written information received in hospital

At the hospital interview, thirteen (22.8%) patients and five (41.7%) carers reported that they had received written information about stroke. Of these thirteen patients, five (38.5%) received one written material, six (46.2 %) received two materials and one (7.7%) each received three and four materials. Of the five carers who received information, one (20%) received two written materials, three (60%) received three materials, and one (20%) received four materials.

Across all participants who received information, thirty-nine pieces of written material were received; twenty-three (59%) by patients, fifteen (38.5%) by carers and one (2.6%) was given jointly to the patient and the carer. Materials consisted of fact sheets and brochures from local (n=9) and national (n=12) stroke associations and the hospital's allied health departments (n=9), and exercise sheets from the stroke unit therapists (n=9). The reported source of the written information was:

- patient or carer picked it up from the stroke unit bookshelf (nineteen pieces of material; 48.7%)
- provided by the stroke unit speech pathologist (eleven pieces of material; 28.2%)
- provided by the occupational therapist (seven pieces of material; 17.9%)
- provided by the dietician (one piece of material; 2.6%)
- provided by the physiotherapist (one piece of material; 2.6%).

Of the thirty-nine pieces of material received by participants, thirty-one pieces (79.5%) were reported to be read. The reasons given for not reading them were: material considered too long

($n=1$); preference for reading the information when discharged home ($n=3$); received too soon after stroke ($n=1$); not yet had time to read it ($n=2$); and forgotten that it had been received ($n=1$).

Written information received after discharge

At the six-month interview, only three (6.1%) of the forty-nine patients interviewed at follow-up had received written information about stroke since the initial interview. The source of this information was a family member who had printed it from the internet ($n=1$) and an occupational therapist ($n=1$) and speech pathologist ($n=1$) in outpatient rehabilitation. Materials consisted of a speech pathology department brochure, an information kit from the local stroke association and a fact sheet from a website about atrial fibrillation. All three pieces of information were reported to be read.

Satisfaction with information received

Participants' mean satisfaction score with the content of the written information received was 9.0 (standard deviation$=1.4$, range$=5$–10) and 9.3 (standard deviation$=1.34$, range$=4$–10) for presentation. The most frequently reported positive features of the written information were:

- the information explained things
- it was easy to understand
- it had helpful pictures
- it gave practical information.

The most frequently reported negative features were:

- the font was too small
- it was hard to understand
- it contained irrelevant information.

Informational needs

At the hospital interview, twenty-three (40.4%) patients and eight (66.7%) carers had unanswered questions about stroke, including:

- the reason for the cause of the stroke (n=14)
- questions about recovery from stroke (n=9)
- the chance of having another stroke (n=6)

- how to prevent further strokes (n=4)
- an explanation for jargon/abbreviations (eg. TIA, MRI) (n=3)
- returning to driving (n=3)
- the relationship between stroke and heart attack (n=3)
- the reason for various tests (n=2)
- questions about the severity of the individual's stroke (n=2)
- explanation of the effects of stroke (n=2)
- questions about supports and services available after discharge (n=2).

By follow-up, the number of participants with unanswered questions had decreased to thirteen (26.5%) patients and one (11.1%) carer. The questions that were asked related to recovery after stroke (*n*=7), effects of stroke (*n*=4), medications (*n*=3) and chances of another stroke (*n*=1).

Table 14.2 presents the frequency of participants, at hospital and follow-up interview, who expressed an interest in receiving information about one or more of the pre-identified stroke-related topics. At the hospital interview, nearly all participants — fifty-two (91.2%) patients and twelve (100%) carers — wanted more information about stroke. More than half of the patients wanted more information on such topics as:

- preventing further strokes (77%)
- where to obtain further information (65%)
- causes of stroke (65%)
- risk factors of stroke (61%)
- recovery (60%)
- what a stroke is (54%)
- stroke-related medications (53%).

At least half of the carers also wanted information on these topics. In addition, 75% of carers wanted information about the emotional or psychological effects of stroke. At the follow-up interview, 75.5% of patients and all carers wanted further information. Again, the most frequently desired topic, by both patients and carers, was prevention of further strokes.

Participants had a clear preference for written information at both time-points. Of the fifty-two patients desiring information at the hospital interview, fifty (96.2%) requested written information and one (1.9%) patient each wanted face-to-face discussion with a doctor and a combination of written information and verbal discussion. Eleven (91.7%) of the carers wanted written information and one (8.3%) wanted a combination of written information and verbal discussion.

At follow-up, of the thirty-seven patients desiring additional information, thirty-one (83.8%) expressed a preference for written information, three (8.1%) for talking with rehabilitation therapists and one (2.7%) each for face-to-face talk with a doctor, telephone conversation with a doctor and a combination of written information and verbal discussion. Seven (77.8%) of the carers requested written information and one each (11.1%) preferred a face-to-face conversation with a doctor and a combination of written information and verbal discussion.

Table 14.2: Comparison of participant-identified informational needs at time of hospital interview and six-month follow-up interview

| Topics related to stroke | No. participants who would have liked to receive information about the topic (%) | | | |
| | Hospital interview | | Follow-up interview | |
	Patients (n=57)	Carers (n=12)	Patients (n=49)	Carers (n=9)
What is a stroke?	31 (54%)	6 (50%)	9 (18%)	1 (11%)
Causes of stroke	37 (65%)	8 (67%)	10 (20%)	2 (22%)
Risk factors of stroke	35 (61%)	8 (67%)	11 (22%)	2 (22%)
Treatment available after stroke	27 (47%)	6 (50%)	5 (10%)	0
Recovery after stroke	34 (60%)	6 (50%)	10 (20%)	0
Medications prescribed after a stroke	30 (53%)	6 (50%)	8 (16%)	1 (11%)
Physical effects of stroke	26 (46%)	6 (50%)	5 (10%)	0
Emotional/psychological effects of stroke	24 (42%)	9 (75%)	4 (8%)	1 (11%)
Cognitive effects of stroke	27 (47%)	7 (58%)	12 (24%)	3 (33%)
Communication effects of stroke	17 (30%)	3 (25%)	3 (6%)	1 (11%)
Incontinence following stroke	4 (7%)	3 (25%)	2 (4%)	0
Behavioural effects of stroke	0	1 (8%)	2 (4%)	0
Effects of stroke on family and/or marriage	4 (7%)	2 (17%)	0	2 (22%)
What to expect in rehabilitation	4 (7%)	1 (8%)	n/a	n/a
What to expect at home	21 (37%)	5 (42%)	n/a	n/a
How to prevent further strokes	44 (77%)	10 (83%)	22 (45%)	6 (67%)
Community services available for stroke patients	23 (40%)	6 (50%)	2 (4%)	1 (11%)
Stroke support groups	12 (21%)	2 (17%)	2 (4%)	1 (11%)
Legal information following stroke	6 (11%)	3 (25%)	3 (6%)	1 (11%)
Financial information following stroke (ie, benefits)	7 (12%)	5 (42%)	2 (4%)	0
Equipment and aids necessary after a stroke	13 (23%)	4 (33%)	2 (4%)	0
Information about exercises/activities after a stroke	25 (44%)	2 (17%)	8 (16%)	0
Information about healthy living (eg. tips for exercising)	25 (44%)	3 (25%)	7 (14%)	0
Where to obtain further support/information	37 (65%)	9 (75%)	11 (22%)	3 (33%)
Tips for performing self-care tasks	n/a	n/a	3 (6%)	0
Tips for performing household tasks	n/a	n/a	1 (2%)	0
Returning to community activities	n/a	n/a	1 (2%)	0
Returning to driving	0	0	4 (8%)	0
Helpful tips for carers	0	0	1 (2%)	2 (22%)

n/a = not applicable because these topics were only addressed at one of the interviews

Reading ability scores for participants

At the hospital interview, the mean REALM score for patients was 53.5 (standard deviation=18.2; range=0–66), which equates to a 7th–8th grade reading level (typically equivalent to 12–13 years of age in the Australian education system). Six patients were unable to complete the REALM owing to stroke-related impairments. The mean REALM score for carers was 65.4 (standard deviation=1.1, range=63–66), which is equivalent to a 9th grade or greater reading level. At follow-up, the mean REALM score for patients was 58.5 (standard deviation=13.9, range=0–66), which equates to a 7th–8th grade reading level. One patient was unable to complete the REALM at follow-up.

Readability and suitability of written information received

In total, eighteen of the twenty-two written materials received by participants were analysed. The four materials that were not analysed were handouts illustrating exercises prescribed by the speech pathologist ($n=3$) and physiotherapist ($n=1$).

The mean SMOG readability level of the written materials was equivalent to a grade 11 level of education (standard deviation=1.9, range=8–14). Specifically, 11% were at a grade 8 level equivalent, 11% at grade 9, 28% at grade 11, 28% at grade 12, 6% at grade 13 and 16% at grade 14. Using the Suitability Assessment of Materials checklist, the mean suitability score was 56% (standard deviation=9.9, range=38–71). A total of sixteen (88.9%) of the written materials were rated as adequate, with one (5.6%) each rated as superior and not suitable.

Discussion

The results of this study clearly show that the informational needs of stroke patients and their carers are not being met by current practice. The majority of patients would have liked to receive information about stroke, but only 22% actually did.

These findings concur with other studies that have examined the provision of written materials to stroke patients. Wellwood *et al* (1994) interviewed stroke patients and carers about four weeks after discharge and found that only 12% of patients and 19% of carers had received any written information about stroke and that 53% of patients and 75% of carers would have liked to receive written information. Another study found that at two weeks and at six months after discharge, only 22% and 26% of patients respectively could recall being given written information (Hanger *et al*, 1998).

Almost half of the written information received in this study was collected by the patient or carer from the ward's bookshelf. While having written information freely available for self-collection is convenient, it may not be a satisfactory substitute for the targeted exchange of information from health professional to patient. Ideally, the provision of written information should be accompanied by verbal education (Ley, 1988).

Only three patients reported receiving written information between discharge and the six-month follow-up. Given that stroke is a chronic disease, for which there is a substantial risk of recurrence, the provision of information should not cease at discharge. It may be more appropriate for information to be distributed after discharge, when patients and carers are better able to assimilate information (Greveson and James, 1991) and ask questions about managing any residual effects of stroke.

Unless receiving ongoing outpatient rehabilitation or routine GP follow-up appointments, a large proportion of patients do not have any contact with health professionals after discharge, especially those with neurological expertise. GPs are ideally positioned to be providers of information after discharge, particularly information related to preventing further strokes and questions about medication. Because much information desired by participants was general information about stroke, this could be distributed in written form before discharge via support groups, or made available online.

Most patients identified written information as their preferred method for receiving additional information. This finding may be a result of the short-stay nature of the stroke unit, which may not afford patients or carers an opportunity to establish ongoing relationships with health professionals that will continue after discharge (Greveson and James, 1991). Alternatively, participants may like the fact that written information allows them to absorb the material at their own pace and refer back to it at any time (Bernier, 1993). It is also possible that participants' responses were influenced by their awareness that written information was the focus of this study.

The positive and negative features of the written materials identified by participants in this study are consistent with recommendations in the literature about which features should be incorporated into health education materials (Vahabi and Ferris, 1995; Doak et al, 1996a; Buxton, 1999; Lorig, 2001). Although most participants who received written materials could identify features that they disliked, overall their mean satisfaction scores with the content and presentation of the materials were high. One possible explanation for this, as suggested by participants' comments, is that they preferred to receive some written materials, regardless of the quality. Alternatively, the high satisfaction scores may be a result of participants' unwillingness to criticise services that they felt were helping them. Satisfaction surveys in health care have been found to be prone to such 'response acquiescence' (Keith, 1998).

There are a number of similarities between the results of this study, in terms of patients' informational needs, and the results of two other studies (van Veenendaal et al, 1996; Hanger et al, 1998). Hanger et al examined what patients and carers wanted to know about stroke over a two-year period and found an increased focus on questions about the cognitive and psychological effects of stroke as time since discharge increased. Further, they reported that participants' questions about preventing further strokes remained a continued focus at all three points in time and that there were very few questions about some of the common sequelae of stroke, namely hemiplegia and incontinence. Van Veenendaal et al (1996) also found that patients and family members most desired information about preventing another stroke, closely followed by information about risk factors and causes of stroke.

In the study described in this chapter, there was some improvement in the mean REALM score (ie. reading ability) for patients over time. This has implications for the provision of written materials while patients are in hospital. First, the readability level of materials provided while in hospital may need to be lower than that of materials given after discharge. The neurological deficits that occur with stroke, such as aphasia, unilateral neglect and hemianopia can affect reading ability and their impact may be greater during the acute phase. Second, to enhance understanding of the information, health professionals may routinely need to supplement the written material with verbal explanation.

The reading grade level of all of the received materials is substantially higher than the maximum grade 6 reading level that is recommended for all health-related materials (Fisher, 1999) and higher than participants' mean reading ability.

Limitations

A number of limitations of this study should be acknowledged. This study was limited to one metropolitan hospital and results may not be generalisable to other settings. The provision of written materials was assessed through self-report and it is possible that some participants might not have recalled receiving written materials, particularly between discharge and the six-month interview. There were some carers who were unable to participate in the follow-up interview and some who were not present for the hospital interview, which limited the extent to which change in carers' needs and reading abilities could be examined.

Conclusion

This study supports previous findings that stroke patients and carers want substantially more information than they are receiving, both while in hospital and six months later. Health professionals working with stroke patients need to assess routinely and meet the informational needs of their patients and be attentive to the issues surrounding the provision of written information. These issues include when and how the information should be provided, ensuring that the patient is aware of methods for receiving information after discharge, and that when providing written information, issues such as readability and suitability, along with the patient's reading ability, are considered.

References

Bernier MJ (1993) Developing and evaluating printed education materials: a prescriptive model for quality. *Orthop Nurs* **12:** 39–46

Buxton T (1999) Effective ways to improve health education materials. *J Health Educ* **30:** 47–50

Cooper H, Booth K, Fear S, Gill G (2001) Chronic disease patient education: lessons from meta-analyses. *Patient Educ Couns* **44**: 107–17

Doak CC, Doak L, Gordon L, Lorig K (2001) Selecting, preparing and using materials. In: Lorig K (ed) *Patient Education: A Practical Approach*. Sage Publications, California: 183–97

Doak LG, Doak CC, Meade CD (1996a) Strategies to improve cancer education materials. *Oncol Nurs Forum* **23**: 1305–12

Doak CC, Doak L, Root JH (1996b) *Teaching Patients With Low Literacy Skills*. JB Lippincott, Philadelphia

Eames S, McKenna K, Worrall L, Read S (2003) The suitability of written education materials for stroke survivors and their carers. *Top Stroke Rehabil* **10**: 70–83

Estrada CA, Hryniewicz MM, Higgs VB, Collins C, Byrd JC (2000) Anticoagulant patient information material is written at high readability levels. *Stroke* **31**: 2966–70

Evans RL, Matlock A-L, Bishop DS, Stranahan S, Pederson C (1988) Family intervention after stroke: does counselling or education help? *Stroke* **19**: 1243–9

Fisher E (1999) Low literacy levels in adults: implications for patient education. *J Contin Educ Nurs* **30**: 56–61

Greveson G, James O (1991) Improving long-term outcome after stroke — the views of patients and carers. *Health Trends* **23**: 161–2

Hanger H, Walker G, Paterson L, McBride S, Sainsbury R (1998) What do patients and their carers want to know about stroke? A two-year follow-up study. *Clin Rehabil* **12**: 45–52

Jimenez SLM (1994) Evaluating the readability of written patient education materials. *J Perinatal Educ* **3**: 59–62

Keith R (1998) Patient satisfaction and rehabilitation services. *Arch Phys Med Rehabil* **79**: 1122–8

Ley P (1988) *Communicating With Patients. Improving Communication, Satisfaction and Compliance*. Chapman & Hall, London

Lorig K (2001) *Patient Education — a Practical Approach*. Sage Publications, California

McLaughlin H (1969) SMOG grading: a new readability formula. *J Reading* **12**: 639–46

Murphy PW, Davis TC, Long SW, Jackson RH, Decker BC (1993) Rapid Estimate of Adult Literacy in Medicine (REALM): a quick reading test for patients. *J Reading* **37**: 124–30

O'Mahoney PG, Rodgers H, Thomson RG, Dobson R, James OF (1997) Satisfaction with information and advice received by stroke patients. *Clin Rehabil* **11**: 68–72

Sullivan K, O'Conor F (2001) A readability analysis of Australian stroke information. *Top Stroke Rehabil* **7**: 52–60

Vahabi M, Ferris L (1995) Improving written patient education materials: a review of the evidence. *Health Educ J* **54**: 99–106

van Veenendaal Hv, Grinspun DR, Adriaanse HP (1996) Educational needs of stroke survivors and their family members, as perceived by themselves and by health professionals. *Patient Educ Couns* **28**: 265–76

Webber GC (1990) Patient education. A review of the issues. *Med Care* **28**: 1089–103

Wellwood I, Dennis M, Warlow C (1994) Perceptions and knowledge of stroke among surviving patients with stroke and their carers. *Age Ageing* **23:** 293–8

Wiles R, Pain H, Buckland S, McLellan L (1998) Providing appropriate information to patients and carers following a stroke. *J Adv Nurs* **28:** 794–80

CHAPTER 15

Education in stroke: strategies to improve stroke patient care

Patrick Gompertz, Andrew Slack, Mira Vogel, Sharon Burrows, Philippa Clark

'Stroke units save lives', but organised care requires expert staff and regular training to be effective. However, the quality of inpatient care for stroke remains poor, and stroke education is often fragmented between the healthcare professions. This chapter describes some national and local strategies aimed at ensuring that all patients are cared for by expert staff.

In 2000, the Intercollegiate Working Party for Stroke recommended that:

> *Every organisation involved in the care of stroke patients over the first six months should ensure that stroke patients are the responsibility of and are seen by services specialising in stroke and rehabilitation. The stroke service should comprise: a geographically identified unit acting as a base, and as part of the inpatient service, a coordinated multidisciplinary team, staff with expertise in stroke and rehabilitation, educational programmes for staff, patients and carers.*
>
> *National Clinical Guidelines for Stroke* (First edition)
> (Royal College of Physicians, 2000)

The focus of this statement is on hospital inpatient services for stroke. However, stroke patients present acutely to a range of specialties and to general practice. The problems patients experience after stroke are dealt with by a wide variety of healthcare and social services professionals and carers in a wide spectrum of settings, ranging from the community, acute hospital wards and geriatric wards to nursing and residential homes. It therefore seems appropriate to propose that, in addition, GPs and other hospital specialists have knowledge of stroke, nursing staff and professions allied to medicine are able to manage stroke, and social workers, home carers and nursing home staff are familiar with stroke-related problems. Only in this way can we be sure that all stroke patients receive treatment and care from expert staff throughout their illness.

This chapter describes some national and local strategies, which hopefully will move us closer to achieving this vision of improved interdisciplinary stroke education, but first it reviews the current situation and describes the low base from which this work starts.

Patrick Gompertz, Andrew Slack, Mira Vogel, Sharon Burrows, Philippa Clark

The problem

Stroke is a major burden on NHS resources, constituting over 4% of NHS expenditure. Stroke is the third highest cause of death in the UK and the biggest single cause of major disability (Martin *et al*, 1988). Despite this, Rudd *et al* (1999) have confirmed that the quality of inpatient care for stroke remains poor, and although stroke is a common condition, it is under-represented in most undergraduate curricula and in the examinations for membership of the royal colleges. Teaching is often fragmented between neurologists, physicians and geriatricians. There is also widespread ignorance about stroke-management among nursing staff and carers in the community.

Interdisciplinary working is a key component of effective stroke care. However, the different disciplines train in isolation, and clinical practice may be influenced by different theoretical perspectives (Lacey, 1998). There is also widespread ignorance among the general public about the signs and symptoms and risk factors for stroke, and the effectiveness of treatment (Pancioli *et al*, 1997). Finally, research in stroke is under-resourced and there are few academics specialising in stroke medicine. Perhaps all this has come about because of previously widespread misconceptions about stroke — for example, that stroke is not amenable to medical treatment; rehabilitation does not involve doctors; stroke can be managed effectively by generalists without specialist expertise; and the neurology of stroke is straightforward.

Drivers for change

Despite these problems, there are some encouraging signs and recent developments, which are grounds for cautious optimism. The *National Service Framework for Older People* (Department of Health [DoH], 2001) devotes a section to stroke applicable to all ages, with a prescription and a timetable for change. The *National Clinical Guidelines for Stroke* (Royal College of Physicians, 2000) and the sentinel audit (Rudd *et al*, 1999) have stimulated a great deal of local developments. The British Association of Stroke Physicians (BASP) has a growing membership and the potential to lobby for change, as well as leading developments in the specialty. The sponsorship of research and teaching by the Stroke Association over the years has been a powerful force in influencing these developments and raising the profile of stroke.

Why is education in stroke important?

Education about the management of stroke involves covering a wide range of important concepts in a modern healthcare system, such as multidisciplinary working, holistic care, rehabilitation and the use of organised services to improve outcome. The Stroke Unit Triallists' Collaboration (2001) found that regular staff training and the level of staff expertise and knowledge were factors that distinguished stroke unit care from routine care. Implicitly, the improved outcomes associated with organised care are, at least in part, a result of staff training. Indredavik *et al* (1999) found that mobilisation therapy on the stroke unit was initiated by nurses and therefore began sooner. This was the result of physiotherapy training. In contrast, on the general wards, delays occurred because mobilisation depended on physiotherapy.

Effective interdisciplinary care requires that nurses, medical staff and therapists understand each others' roles and expertise. Often, understanding is required because roles can become blurred. For example, nurses have the main responsibility for ensuring safe positioning of patients and the greatest opportunity to ensure posture is effectively managed. To do this effectively, communication and understanding between nurses and physiotherapists need to be at a high level. Short, targeted community-awareness programmes can increase knowledge about stroke among potential patients and carers (Stern *et al*, 1999).

What can be done?

Clearly, a wide range of initiatives is needed, and many are already taking place. This chapter will highlight the role of the BASP in promoting the subspecialty of stroke medicine, and describe some local developments as examples of potential approaches to the problem.

Setting-up an interprofessional training programme

A complex area of healthcare such as stroke demands effective interaction between the professionals involved, and there is evidence that interdisciplinary working improves outcomes (Zwarenstein *et al*, 2001a). Interprofessional education (when members of more than one healthcare and/or social care profession learn interactively together) may have the potential to enhance collaborative practice; however, its effectiveness remains to be formally established (Zwarenstein *et al*, 2001b).

A multidisciplinary project team was set up to establish an interprofessional learning programme. The team carried out a training-needs analysis for all professional groups involved in care delivery. The analysis took account of the Intercollegiate Working Party for Stroke's *National Clinical Guidelines for Stroke* (Royal College of Physicians, 2000), standard five of the *National Service Framework for Older People* (DoH, 2001) and the local trust's performance development scheme. Two one-day workshops and two focus groups were used to identify the perceived needs of staff.

As a result of this work, training needs were identified that went beyond the purely clinical components of care specified in the guidelines. Staff needed to know about aspects of the organisation of care, such as the key worker role and the discharge process. Interpersonal skills needed development, especially counselling skills, and managing conflict and challenging behaviour. Time-management skills and leadership were important, as was knowledge of quality issues. Learning outcomes needed to be specified in each of the core areas.

Learning needs were addressed by a combination of approaches. In the first instance, a

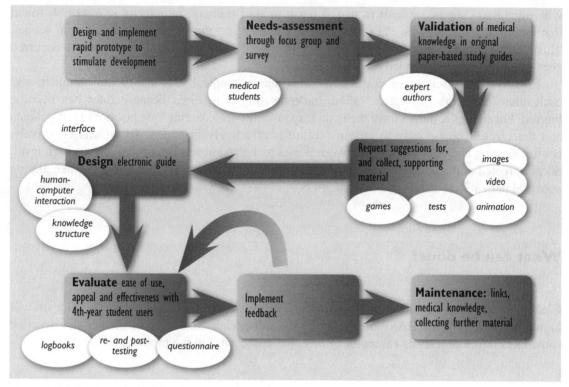

Figure 15.1: Developing a CD-ROM study guide.

basic training programme in stroke was offered to all staff, which covered general anatomy and physiology of stroke, risk factors and prevention, presentation and principles of rehabilitation. Sessions were scheduled to accommodate the maximum number of staff and to coordinate with nursing shift patterns. The purpose of these sessions was to provide all staff with a basic understanding of stroke and a basis on which to build further skills and knowledge.

In addition, it was important to use existing service developments (eg. multidisciplinary task groups to devise new systems of teamworking in the rehabilitation setting) in a way that involved all staff and offered learning opportunities. Also, service-wide workshops (eg. managing challenging behaviour, leadership development, elder abuse workshops) were used for areas not specifically related to stroke. Regular multidisciplinary team meetings were used as learning opportunities.

Teaching methods

According to Thomson O'Brien *et al* (2001), continuing educational meetings containing interactive workshops with or without didactic presentations are moderately effective in changing behaviour — but didactic presentations alone seem to have disappointing results. There has been a great deal of progress in knowledge and structures related to the delivery of educational programmes, which is outside the scope of this chapter. However, the management of stroke as a topic demands the use of the most modern teaching techniques and strategies — for example, problem-based learning, new technology and assessment techniques.

The stroke CD-ROM

The authors have a particular interest in the use of multimedia and other learning aids. As part of a series of study guides (tutorials in print) on medicine in old age, experts at St Bartholomew's Hospital London ('Bart's') and the London Queen Mary's School of Medicine and Dentistry and at the Queen's University Belfast have produced a study guide on stroke. This guide is regularly updated and forms the core of undergraduate training in stroke at both medical schools. Work is ongoing to develop the guide in electronic format, promoting self-paced, active learning and freeing tutorial time for discussion of problem areas.

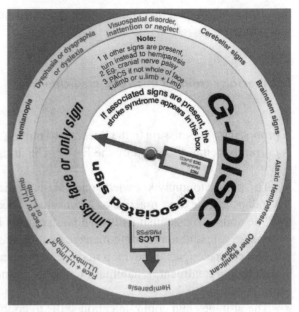

Figure 15.2: The G-disc.

Students have been consulted at all stages of development, and their feedback — in the form of completed questionnaires, logbooks, directed sessions using the study guide and focus-group discussion — continues to guide the expansion of the project. The development process is outlined in *Figure 15.1*.

The G-disc

The Oxford Community Stroke Project (OCSP) classification (Bamford, 1992) is an excellent framework for teaching the neurological assessment and phenomenology of stroke. While it is well-established among stroke physicians, familiarity and regular use of this system has not yet become widespread. This is unfortunate because the system has many advantages for teaching:

- It is comprehensive, including all stroke types, and haemorrhages and infarcts.
- It is clinical rather than based on investigations.
- It carries the important message that all strokes are not the same, and it can be used by non-experts.
- It is also useful to promote an understanding of important concepts, such as localisation of function, so that all staff can differentiate, say, confusion from dysphasia.

Walsh *et al* (2000) have developed a diagnostic and teaching tool based on the OCSP classification. The G-disc is constructed from three separate wheels made of laminate or card (*Figure 15.2*). The user is prompted to look for neurological findings that discriminate between the stroke subtypes. Pilot studies have demonstrated its validity and reliability, and it is popular with students.

Subspecialty training in stroke medicine

A proposal for submission to the Specialist Training Authority for a subspecialty of stroke medicine is currently being discussed by the BASP. The aims of the proposed training are to promote:

- The ability to apply knowledge and skills in diagnosis and management to ensure safe and independent expert practice as a consultant specialist in stroke medicine.
- The ability to establish a differential diagnosis in the context of stroke presentations to ensure safe and appropriate management of acute stroke and non-stroke illness.
- The competencies to develop management plans for people living with stroke illness including treatment, rehabilitation, health promotion, secondary prevention and long-term support.
- The attitudes and communication skills to contribute to a comprehensive multidisciplinary stroke service in hospital and/or the community and to work closely with other relevant agencies.
- The understanding to work effectively within a multidisciplinary stroke service.
- The abilities to advise, develop and evaluate district stroke services in partnership with local health and social care communities.

Conclusion

Stroke medicine is an exciting and expanding field, which is important for a wide range of medical professionals, nursing staff, healthcare staff and professionals allied to medicine. At the moment, the national level of stroke expertise is limited, and it is important that those with expertise should vocally implement strategies to share their skills and knowledge with as many of the relevant groups as possible. The success with which they do this will to a large extent determine local ability to meet Government standards. The creation of an accredited subspecialty stroke training programme is an interesting approach, the implications of which need to be explored.

Conflict of interest: Dr P Gompertz received an educational grant to support the development of the G-disc from Boehringer Ingelheim.

References

Bamford J (1992) Clinical examination in the diagnosis and subclassification of stroke. *Lancet* **339**: 400–2

DoH (2001) *National Service Framework for Older People*. DoH, London

Indredavik B, Slordahl S, Haheim L (1999) Treatment in a combined acute and rehabilitation stroke unit: which aspects are most important? *Stroke* **30**: 917–23

Intercollegiate Working Party for Stroke (2000) *National Clinical Guidelines for Stroke*. Royal College of Physicians, London

Lacey P (1998) Interdisciplinary training for staff working with people with profound and multiple learning difficulties. *J Interprofessional Care* **12**(1): 43–52

Martin J, Meltzer H, Elliot D (1988) OPCS surveys of disability in Great Britain Report 1. In: *The Prevalence of Disability Among Adults*. Office of Population Censuses and Surveys. HMSO, London

Pancioli A, Broderick J, Kothari R, Brott T, Khoury J, Liu T (1997) Patients' awareness of stroke signs, symptoms and risk factors. *Stroke* **28**: 1871–5

Rudd AG, Irwin P, Rutledge Z *et al* (1999) The national sentinel audit of stroke: a tool for raising standards of care. *J R Coll Physicians Lond* **33**: 460–4

Stern E, Berman M, Thomas J, Klassen A (1999) Community education for stroke awareness. *Stroke* **30**: 720–3

Stroke Unit Triallists' Collaboration (2001) Organised inpatient (stroke unit) care for stroke (Cochrane review). In: The Cochrane Library. Issue 2. Update Software, Oxford

Thomson O'Brien MA, Fremantel N, Oxman AD, Wolf F, Davis DA, Herrin J (2001) Continuing education meetings and workshops: effects on professional practice and healthcare outcomes (Cochrane review). In: The Cochrane Library. Issue 2. Update Software, Oxford

Walsh K, Gompertz P, Chen P, Cawley C (2000) Preliminary evaluation of a diagnostic disc in the classification of stroke syndromes. *Age Ageing* **29**(suppl 2): 53

Zwarenstein M, Bryant W (2001a) Interventions to promote collaboration between nurses and doctors (Cochrane review). In: The Cochrane Library. Issue 2. Update Software, Oxford

Zwarenstein M, Reeves S, Barr H, Hammick M, Koppel I, Atkins J (2001b) Interprofessional education: effects on professional practice and health care outcomes (Cochrane review). In: The Cochrane Library. Issue 2. Update Software, Oxford

CHAPTER 16

Cognitive impairments following a stroke: the strain on caregivers

Holly Blake, Nadina B Lincoln

This chapter aims to investigate the relation between cognitive impairment in stroke patients and strain in their spouses. The condition was assesssed in patients from stroke wards and general medical wards in four acute general hospitals and its impact on caregivers was analysed.

Patients with hemispheric stroke have a combination of motor, sensory and cognitive impairments (Lezak, 1983). Cognitive deficits may include impairments of memory, language or perception, or cognitive impairments such as reasoning difficulties. Specific cognitive deficits affect the rehabilitation process and are likely to be a major barrier to independence (Jongbloed, 1986).

The National Strategy for Carers (Department of Health [DoH], 1998) outlined the importance of supporting caregivers for the benefit of both caregiver and care-receiver, and claimed that:

> *better-supported carers will be able to make better lives for the people for whom they care.*

The early identification of carers who may be unable to cope later after stroke would enable effective targeting of support to prevent carer strain. Previous research has suggested that characteristics of the carer are more important in determining the level of strain experienced by them than mood or disability of the patient (Blake and Lincoln, 2000). However, studies assessing patient characteristics are often limited to biographical characteristics and measures of activities of daily living (ADL) and do not address the impact of stroke on cognitive function.

The impact of patient cognitive impairment on the caregiver is unclear. A study of carer burden after proximal femoral fracture found that carers of patients who were cognitively impaired on the Short Portable Mental Status Questionnaire (Pfeiffer, 1975) suffered from higher levels of burden than carers of patients who were not (Quine *et al*, 1994; Drinka *et al*, 1987) linked caregiver burden and depression to cognitive impairment in patients attending a geriatric referral clinic, as measured on the Jacobs Cognitive Capacity Screening Exam (Jacobs *et al*, 1977).

Few studies have been identified in which cognitive deficits have been examined in relation to strain in spouses of stroke patients. An early study by Kinsella and Duffy (1979) found that spouses of aphasic stroke patients had poorer overall social adjustment and a higher incidence of minor psychiatric disorder than spouses of non-aphasic patients. Perceptual problems may interfere with ADL and quality of life for the patient, which may have an effect on the spouse. A deficit of executive function may cause difficulties in reasoning, planning ahead and making decisions (Lezak, 1983). It is not unreasonable to hypothesise that this may impact on the quality of life for both the patient and the spouse. The aim of this study was to determine the relationship between cognitive deficit of the stroke patient and caregiver strain.

Method

Patients

This study was a secondary analysis of data collected as part of a single-blind randomised controlled trial evaluating the impact of cognitive assessment in multidisciplinary stroke rehabilitation (McKinney *et al*, 2001). In this trial, patients who suffered strokes according to the World Health Organisation (WHO) (1978) definition were recruited from four hospitals within four weeks of admission. Patients and carers giving informed consent were considered for inclusion provided the patient was not unconscious on admission (as assessed on a four-point scale of 'unconscious', 'semi-

Table 16.1: Distibution of patient characteristics

Patient chacteristic		n (%)
Centre	Nottingham	63 (49)
	Derby	46 (35)
	Mansfield	21 (16)
Hospital	UHN	63 (49)
	DCGH	33 (25)
	DRI	13 (10)
	MCH	21 (16)
Level of consciousness	Alert	98 (75)
	Drowsy	18 (14)
	Semi-conscious	6 (5)
	Unknown	8 (6)
Side of weakness affected	Left	65 (50)
	Right	57 (44)
	No lateralised weakness	8(6)
Swallowing difficulties	Difficulties	48 (37)
	No difficulties	76 (58)
	Unknown	6 (5)
Incontinence of bladder	Continent	73 (56)
	Incontinent	52 (40)
	Unknown	5 (4)
Incontinence of bowels	Continent	95 (73)
	Incontinent	29 (22)
	Unknown	6 (5)
Weakness in arm	No deficit	7 (5)
	Weakness	105 (81)
	No movement	15 (12)
	Unknown	3 (2)
Weakness in leg	No deficit	13 (10)
	Weakness	108 (83)
	No movement	6 (5)
	Unknown	3 (2)

DCGH=Derby City General Hospital; DRI=Derby Royal Infirmary; MCH=Mansfield Community Hospital; UHN=University Hospital Nottingham

conscious', 'drowsy' or 'alert'), could sit and cooperate with the assessments for thirty minutes at a time and had no significant visual and hearing impairments preventing them from completing the screening battery.

Biographical characteristics, pre-stroke Barthel Index (Collin *et al*, 1988), Barthel Index at time of recruitment and details of stroke were also recorded.

Procedure

All recruited patients were assessed on a screening battery by an assistant psychologist to determine the presence of cognitive problems. The screening battery included the Mini-Mental State Examination (MMSE) (Folstein *et al*, 1975), the Sheffield Screening Test for Acquired Language Disorders (SST) (Syder *et al*, 1993) and Raven's Coloured Progressive Matrices (RCPM) (Raven, 1965). Used as a non-verbal assessment of intelligence, the RCPM is based on visual perceptual abilities and analogical reasoning. Two scores were used: the number correct score as a measure of non-verbal reasoning and the proportion of right:left responses as a measure of visual inattention. Caregiver strain on the Caregiver Strain Index (CSI) (Robinson, 1983) was measured three and six months after admission to the ward.

Results

A total of 228 stroke patients were recruited, of whom 162 (71%) patients identified a main carer and of these, 130 were spouses. There were eighty-three male and forty-seven female stroke patients with spouses. Patient ages ranged from twenty-nine to eighty-nine years (mean=68.33, standard deviation [sd]=11.46). Mean pre-stroke Barthel Index was 19.37 (sd=1.78) and mean Barthel score at time of recruitment was 10.16 (sd=5.94). The distribution of patient characteristics is shown in *Table 16.1*.

Table 16.2: Descriptive results for the screening assessments

Assessment	Ability	n	Possible range	Median	IQR
MMSE	General intellectual ability	130	0–30	24	17–27
SST	Expressive skills	129*	0–11	10	7–10
	Receptive skills	129*	0–9	7	5–8
	Aphasia (total score)	129*	0–20	16	11–18
RCPM	Non-verbal reasoning	127**	0–36	19.5	13–26
	Visual neglect	129*	–100–100	0	–7–21

On all tests, higher scores indicate better cognitive function. IQR=inter-quartile range; MMSE=Mini-Mental State Examination; RCPM=Raven's Coloured Progressive Matrices; SST=Sheffield Screening Test for Acquired Language Disorders. *One patient refused to complete the test. **One patient refused to complete the test; two patients were unable to finish the test

Table 16.3: Comparisons of levels of strain according to patient characteristics

Patient characteristic	3 months CSI		6 months CSI	
	n	P	n	P
Gender	71	0.55	74.0	0.46
Group (A/B)	71	0.23	74.0	0.37
Side of weakness	61	0.35	74.0	0.55
Previous stroke	71	0.90	74.0	0.44
Level of consciousness	65	0.41	67.0	0.26
Swallowing difficulties	71	0.29	74.0	0.60
Incontinence of bladder	66	0.78	69.0	0.50
Incontinence of bowel	66	0.37	69.0	0.63

A=screen tests only; B=detailed assessment intervention as part of a randomised controlled trial;
CSI=Caregiver Strain Index

All patients completed the screening assessments. Of these, there were seventy-one whose spouses completed the CSI at three months, and seventy-four whose spouses completed the CSI at six months. Of the fifty-six spouses with no outcome at three months, two were too ill to assess, nine had died, twelve refused follow-up and thirty-six agreed to be involved in the study but then failed to return the CSI. At six months, one patient was too ill to assess and eleven patients had died. Descriptive results for the screening assessments are shown in *Table 16.2*.

Cronbach's alpha for the CSI was 0.80 at three months and 0.81 at six months, indicating good internal consistency. Median CSI was 5 at three months (IQR=2–8) and 5 at six months (IQR=1–8). A Wilcoxin test showed no significant change in strain in the spouse ($z=-1.08$, $P=0.28$). Spouses who scored equal to or greater than seven on the CSI were considered to be under significant strain (Robinson, 1983). Strain at three months was evident in 37% of carers while 34% of carers were strained at six months.

To examine the relationship between early patient characteristics and later strain, Spearman correlation co-efficients were calculated between patients' age, pre-stroke Barthel Index, Barthel Index at recruitment and the CSI. Carers of younger patients reported significantly greater levels of strain at three months than those of older patients ($r^s=-0.33$, $P=0.005$), although age was not related to strain at six months after stroke ($r^s=-0.14$, $P=0.23$). There were no significant relationships between strain and patient independence on the Barthel Index.

Levels of strain were compared between patients with and without the following characteristics using Mann–Whitney U tests or Kruskal–Wallis tests:

- level of consciousness on admission (alert/drowsy/semi-conscious)
- continence of bladder and bowel on admission (yes/no)
- swallowing difficulties on admission (yes/no)
- side of stroke (left/right)
- previous stroke (yes/no)
- gender (male/female)
- weakness in arm and leg (no deficit/weakness/no movement)

- recruitment hospital (Derby City General Hospital, Derby Royal Infirmary, Mansfield Community Hospital, University Hospital, Nottingham)
- recruitment centre (Nottingham, Derby, Mansfield).

Results are shown in *Table 16.3*. There were no significant differences in strain according to the characteristics compared.

Spearman correlation co-efficients were also calculated between each of the cognitive assessments and caregiver strain. Results are shown in *Table 16.4*. General intellectual ability on the MMSE was significantly related to strain at three and six months after stroke. Strain at three months was associated with overall language deficit but this relationship was not maintained at six months. Visual neglect and reasoning on the RCPM were not significantly related to strain. Partial correlation controlling for the effects of age showed no significant relationship between MMSE and caregiver strain at either three months ($r^s=-0.24$, $P=0.08$) or six months ($r^s=-0.13$, $P=0.34$). Additionally, no significant relationship was found between MMSE and caregiver strain at either three months ($r^s=-0.001$, $P=0.99$) or six months ($r^s=-0.08$, $P=0.58$) when the effects of language difficulty were taken into account.

Discussion

Carers of younger patients suffered from a greater level of strain than those of older patients early on after stroke. This finding is consistent with other studies, eg. in a study of informal carers in palliative care (Payne *et al*, 1999), younger age was found to be significantly correlated with strain on the CSI. Level of ability of the patients in basic self-care both before and after the stroke, patient characteristics and impairments did not determine whether the spouses suffered from strain or not.

Spouses of patients whose general intellectual state was poor on the MMSE suffered from increased levels of strain. However, when the effects of age and aphasia were controlled, this relationship was no longer significant. Language deficits were related to increased strain early

Table 16.4: Correlations between cognitive assessments and caregiver strain

Assessment	Ability	CSI at 3 months			CSI at 6 months		
		n	*r^s*	*P*	*n*	*r^s*	*P*
MMSE	General intellectual	71.0	−0.25	0.03*	74.0	−0.24	0.04*
SST	Expressive skills	71.0	−0.23	0.06	74.0	−0.11	0.36
	Reflective skills	71.0	−0.20	0.10	74.0	−0.17	0.15
	Aphasia (total skills)	71.0	−0.25	0.03*	74.0	−0.18	0.14
RCPM	Non-verbal reasoning	71.0	0.09	0.48	74.0	−0.15	0.19
	Visual neglect	71.0	−0.04	0.77	74.0	0.02	0.85

*Significant at $P=0.05$; r^s=correlation co-efficient; CSI=Caregiver Strain Index; MMSE= Mini-Mental State Examination; RCPM=Raven's Coloured Progressive Matrices; SST=Sheffield Screening Test for Acquired Language Disorders

after stroke, but not later. This could be because of the fact that many patients with milder difficulties improved with time. Initial difficulties may have improved by six months after the stroke, thus reducing strain in the spouses by this time. In addition, spouses may have learned to cope with the communication difficulty or received help from speech and language therapists (SLTs) and support groups.

Visual neglect and non-verbal reasoning were not related to strain, suggesting that perception and executive function were not important factors in the level of strain experienced. Acquired perceptual problems are often amenable to treatment and treatment gains can lead to improvements in daily functioning. Slight perceptual deficits may persist, but as patients learn to compensate for these impairments, they may not impact significantly on the well-being of the spouse. It seems that impairments of perception represent less of a strain to the spouse than an inability to communicate with their partner.

The present study suggested that younger age and language deficit were related to strain early after stroke, but later, age appeared to be less important. Although caregiver characteristics were not assessed in this study, our previous work has suggested that caregiver characteristics may play a more important role in the experience of caregiver strain than patient characteristics (Blake and Lincoln, 2000).

As patient numbers were low, univariate analysis was used and therefore no conclusions can be drawn as to how different factors interact with each other and influence caregiver strain in combination. Cognitive function is a complex issue and further studies on larger samples may provide greater insights. Additionally, in clinical practice, a combination of tests might be employed to diagnose a deficit in a particular cognitive function. This might provide more information than simply saying whether a patient was impaired or not on a single neuropsychological test. Nevertheless, it would seem that language is the impairment likely to have most impact on carers and that isolated cognitive impairments may be less important than general cognitive decline.

Conclusion

In this sample, communication difficulties were most likely to affect strain early after stroke. Assessment of specific areas of cognitive deficit including visual neglect and reasoning revealed that impairment of these areas of cognitive function was not related to strain. This suggests that strain in spouses may be related to characteristics other than the cognitive sequalae of stroke.

This research was funded by the Stroke Association. The authors would like to thank the participating patients and carers; Karen Treece and Michelle McKinney for help with data collection and University Hospital, Nottingham, Derby City General Hospital, Derby Royal Infirmary and Mansfield Community Hospital for access to the stroke registers.

References

Blake H, Lincoln NB (2000) Factors associated with strain in co-resident spouses of stroke patients. *Clin Rehabil* **14**(3): 307–14

Collin C, Wade DT, Davis S, Horne V (1988) The Barthel Index: a reliability study. *Int J Disabil Stud* **10**(2): 61–3

DoH (1998) *National Strategy for Carers*. DoH, London

Drinka TJK, Smith JC, Drinka PJ (1987) Correlates of depression and burden for informal caregivers in a geriatric referral clinic. *J Am Geriatrics Soc* **35**: 522–5

Folstein MF, Folstein SE, McHugh PR (1975) Mini-Mental State: a practical method of grading the cognitive status of patients for the clinicians. *J Psychiat Res* **12**: 189–98

Jacobs JW, Bernhard M, Deigado A (1977) Screening for organic mental syndromes in the medically ill. *Annals Int Med* **1**: 40

Jongbloed L (1986) Prediction of function after stroke: a critical review. *Stroke* **17**: 65–76

Kinsella GJ, Duffy FD (1979) Psychosocial readjustment in the spouses of aphasic patients: a comparative survey of seventy-nine subjects. *Scand J Rehabil Med* **11**: 129–32

Lezak MD (1983) *Neuropsychological Assessment*. Oxford University Press, New York

McKinney M, Blake H, Treece KA, Lincoln NB, Playford ED, Gladman JRF (2001) Evaluation of cognitive assessment in stroke rehabilitation. *Clin Rehabil* **16**(2): 129–36

Payne S, Smith P, Dean S (1999) Identifying the concerns of informal carers in palliative care. *Palliative Med* **13**: 37–44

Pfeiffer E (1975) A short portable mental status questionnaire for the assessment of organic brain deficit in elderly patients. *J Am Geriatrics Soc* **23**: 433–41

Quine S, Helby L, Cameron I, Lyle D (1994) Carer burden after proximal femoral fracture. *Disabil Rehabil* **16**(4): 191–7

Raven JC (1965) *Guide to Using the Coloured Progressive Matrices*. HK Lewis, London

Robinson BC (1983) Validation of a caregiver strain index. *J Gerontol* **38**: 344–8

Syder D, Body R, Parker M, Boddy M (1993) *Sheffield Screening Test for Acquired Language Disorders*. NFER-NELSON, Windsor

WHO (1978) *Cerebrovascular Disease: a Clinical And Research Classification. WHO Offset Series No. 34*. WHO, Geneva

CHAPTER 17

Community support after stroke: patient and carer views

Christopher McKevitt, Charles Wolfe

Trials of interventions to support stroke patients and their carers in the community have had disappointing results. Service-user views are accorded increasing importance, but few community stroke interventions have sought the views of potential users about what kinds of support they would wish to see. We report findings from a qualitative study that asked stroke patients and carers to identify the main problems they faced and what they thought a stroke-specific community service should offer. The findings were used to inform the content of a new intervention to be evaluated by randomised controlled trial.

Introduction

The practical, social and emotional problems of stroke survivors discharged home have been long recognised (Holbrook, 1982) and there is a growing body of literature documenting experiences of life after stroke from the perspectives of both survivors and family members/carers (McKevitt *et al*, 2004). The increased recognition of the longer-term consequences of stroke provided the impetus to develop strategies to support survivors and their families in their own homes after the initial acute period of clinical care.

A number of interventions using different approaches have now been evaluated. A US intervention led by social support therapists aimed to improve stroke survivors' psychosocial outcomes by providing improved social support (Friedland and McColl, 1992). In the UK, there have been trials of community support provided by specialist nurses (Forster and Young, 1996), social workers (Dennis *et al*, 1997) and Stroke Association family support organisers (Mant *et al*, 2000; Lincoln *et al*, 2003). Results from these trials have shown few and variable positive effects, or have been inconclusive. For example, Friedland and McColl (1992) found no statistically significant differences between the control and intervention groups in either social support or psychosocial outcomes. Forster and Young (1996) reported no benefits for carers and a moderate increase in social activities in patients with mild disability. Interventions in Edinburgh and Birmingham found no benefits for patients but psychosocial benefits and increased satisfaction with information among carers (Dennis *et al*, 1997; Mant *et al*, 2000). Lincoln *et al* (2003) reported increased knowledge about stroke and services among patients and carers and increased satisfaction with information but no other benefits. Thus, the ability of

Table 17.1: Interview topic guide
The stroke event
Preparation for discharge from the hospital
The experience of returning home
Support received: sources; gaps
A community stroke service: a good idea? What should it offer?

community support services to improve outcomes for people with stroke and those who care for them has not been adequately demonstrated, although some of this uncertainty may arise from methodological considerations. These include the evaluation method used (see, for example, the alternative conclusions reached by Dowswell *et al* [1997] following their qualitative evaluation of a nurse-led intervention), the use of inappropriate outcome measures (Bisset and Chesson, 1997), or the interpretation offered by researchers (Pound *et al*, 1997). Equally, poor results might reflect the inappropriateness of the services themselves.

The importance of consulting users in the development and audit of services has been increasingly recognised (Avis, 1997). In the UK, as elsewhere, user involvement in the planning of health services has become enshrined in Government policy (UK Health and Social Care Act, 2001). It has been argued that such involvement leads to: better-quality and more responsive services; better outcomes of care and better health for the population; reductions in health inequalities; greater local ownership of health services; and a better understanding of why and how local services need to change and develop (www.doh.gov.uk). Yet recent reviews have also suggested that good evidence of the impact of user involvement is still lacking (Crawford *et al*, 2002; Simpson and House, 2002).

At the same time, the UK Medical Research Council has proposed a framework for the development of complex interventions to be evaluated by randomised controlled trial, which incorporates a theoretical phase during which research aimed to inform the development of the intervention should be undertaken (Medical Research Council, 2000). However, it is not clear that community support services for stroke survivors and their families have explicitly sought their views and used these to design the intervention, so it may be that the services do not meet the needs of stroke families, as they perceive them to be.

When our research group undertook to implement and evaluate a community intervention for stroke families, we had unanswered questions about the content and delivery of community support services, as well as outcomes that should be measured in evaluations of such services. We were funded to evaluate a family support organiser (FSO) scheme that was being newly established in a town in southern England. The FSO service is organised by the voluntary sector organisation, the Stroke Association, and may be requested and purchased by primary care trusts. It offers information, emotional support and prevention advice for families and stroke patients, and is aimed to cover the gap in support when formal treatment or therapy ends. Using the approach promoted in the MRC framework for complex interventions (Medical Research Council, 2000), we conducted preliminary research that aimed to define and modify the content of the intervention and identify the most relevant outcomes This entailed a survey of providers of the FSO service nationally to investigate what was provided and how delivery of services was organised (Pound and Wolfe,

Table 17.2: Formal support received

Patient number	Age	Sex	Social class*	Barthel index**	Seen by social worker in hospital	OT home visit	Received written information	Home service	DSG/SA	Day centre	District/diabetes nurse	Respite care
1	79	F	IV	11	Yes			Home help				
2	67	M	V	9	Yes	Yes			Yes	Yes		
3	72	F	II	20		Yes						
4	84	F	IIIM	16	Yes			Carer	Yes			Yes
5	70	F	IIIM	20								
6	61	F	IIIN	20			Yes				Yes	
7	65	M	I	20	Yes	Yes			Yes			
8	73	F	IIIM	19	Yes		Yes					
9	83	F	IIIM	12	Yes	Yes	Yes		Yes	Yes	Yes	
10	87	F	I	20	Yes							
11	71	F	II	20				Cleaner*				
12	72	M	IV	12	Yes		Yes	Bathing		Yes		Yes
13	92	F	IIIM	16								Yes
14	85	M	II	19		Yes						
15	78	F	IIIM	19	Yes			Carer			Yes	
16	71	M	IIIM	17	Yes			Carer				
17	80	F	IV	13	Yes					Yes		Yes
18	84	M	IIIM	19	Yes		Yes					
19	67	M	IIIM	18		Yes						
20	82	M	I	13	Yes		Yes		Yes		Yes	

Blank space signifies 'No'. *Privately purchased; *=social class is based on occupation (usually last job). It was measured using the Standard Occupational Classification produced by the Office of Population Censuses and Surveys. According to occupation, individuals are categorised into 1 of 5 groups, ranging from professional occupations (I) to unskilled occupations (V). **=the Barthel index is a widely used rating scale that assesses functional independence and disability. Domains measured include tasks such as dressing, feeding, walking and toileting. Scores range from 0 (totally dependent) to 20 (totally independent).

1998) and a qualitative interview study with stroke survivors and their carers. In this chapter, we report findings from the latter study, which asked interviewees to identify the main problems they faced and to give their views of what a stroke-specific community service should offer.

Methods

The study took place in the town where the intervention is to be established. We used a qualitative method, since our aim was to allow people to describe their own experiences, perceptions and values (Pope and Mays, 1995), rather than quantifying responses to predetermined categories.

Interviewees were recruited using discharge data from the local district general hospital. We used a purposive sampling method (Fitzpatrick and Boulton, 1994) to select interviewees who varied in terms of age, gender, stroke severity and whether living alone or not. Patients living outside the study area, in residential care prior to the stroke, or with severe speech or cognitive impairments that would make interviewing difficult, were excluded. Selection took place in two stages with the second wave following a review of the first ten interviews. In all, twenty-six people were contacted of whom four did not respond and two declined to participate.

Open-ended interviews were used to allow participants to describe their own experiences in context and raise issues of concern to them. A topic guide was used (*Table 17.1*). Data were also collected about social class, living arrangements and disability (Barthel Index). The interviews lasted forty-five to ninety minutes and were conducted by a social scientist in the patient's or carer's home. They were tape-recorded with consent. Ten interviews were conducted six months after the stroke; six at seven to nine months; and four at ten months. The interviews were transcribed in full, with transcripts analysed using content analysis. This entails reading each transcript; coding text; sorting and re-sorting coded units into thematic categories; and identifying patterns and negative cases. Responses are enumerated to indicate the frequency of themes in this sample.

Findings

Eight interviews were conducted with patients alone and eight with patient and spouse (in one case, the patient's adult son also participated). As four people were, variously, in hospital, in respite care, or unwilling to be interviewed at the time arranged, these interviews were conducted with the patient's adult daughters. *Table 17.2* shows the characteristics of the discharged patient at time of interview. The age of family members interviewed ranged from twenty-nine to eighty-seven years (median sixty-five).

Unanswered questions: what's normal after stroke?

Eleven participants wanted more information about the causes of stroke, implications for future health, and likely prognoses. Carers spoke of their uncertainty about the 'normal' consequences of stroke, and, as one woman said of her husband, what to expect about 'the way he would react and the way I should respond.'

Those who said they did not have unanswered questions were either satisfied with the information they had received or emphasised their own self-confidence, which allowed them to ask for information. One stroke survivor said that he had no unanswered questions as he was more concerned about caring for his wife, and another health problem he had at the time. One woman resisted discussing her stroke with the interviewer, explaining that for her this was a potential cause of stress, something that she now tried to avoid, convinced this was the cause of her stroke.

These differences also reflected individuals' experiences of getting information. Two carers complained that hospital staff did not communicate with them; others acknowledged that doctors and nurses had limited time available for individuals. Five people reported that they were not involved in discharge planning and seven were not aware of any follow-up plan having been made. Yet others were satisfied with the way they had been prepared for discharge, and several recalled a professional (eg. social worker, occupational therapist) who assisted at discharge or assured that they would be available in the future if needed. The style of the contact as much as the content was important, with 'sensitivity' and 'kindness' appreciated.

Practical support at home

Overwhelmingly, people identified family as important sources of practical help, but participants also used a wide range of formal services (*Table 17.2*). Fewer participants than expected identified unmet service needs. One wanted more information about home care and two wanted help with benefits applications. Two carers did not know how to organise respite care, while another was unable to pay the required contribution to the cost of respite care. However, complaints about the slowness of getting aids and adaptations were common. Two interviewees' accounts suggest that they felt overwhelmed by the professional support which was organised or offered.

On-going clinical care

Eight people, including two patients classified as functionally independent (Barthel Index=20) felt that they or the person they cared for had received insufficient physiotherapy, and one insufficient speech therapy. Two people acknowledged that physiotherapists did not agree that further therapy was warranted but felt that a programme of exercises would nevertheless be beneficial Yet others felt that been physiotherapy had been denied or limited because of the patient's age, or for economic reasons. One man, for example, said:

> *That's the only gripe I've got about it all: that I was missing treatment I could have had. It's — they run out of money — they couldn't afford to treat me anymore. You know how it is this day and age... if we'd had more physio', we would've been happier.*
>
> (Interview 12)

Contact with general practice services was reported in seventeen interviews. In nine cases, this was for repeat prescriptions, monitoring, routine checks or other health problems, while three people consulted their GP about affective disorders. However, four people were unhappy with the lack of on-going medical care. For example, one felt that she ought to have her blood pressure monitored, since hypertension had been newly diagnosed and therapy initiated. Others complained more generally about a lack of 'supervision', with one carer explaining:

> Well, the only help that was offered was shopping, housework, and I could cope with that, but I just hope that there will be more supervision of my husband... to make sure that he is making progress.

> (Interview 19)

Emotional and psychological problems

Eleven people reported experiencing some form of emotional problem, including carers who wanted to talk about the fear and frustration that their partner's illness created. They related their distress to the difficulty of getting information about illness trajectories after stroke. However, of these eleven, six said professionals or family and friends had helped them overcome their problems. Another identified the time of her husband's stroke and hospitalisation as the period when she most needed support, and that by the time of the interview she had 'got used to it'. The accounts of two respondents suggest that although they may have had some emotional problems, they did not feel that formal help for such problems was appropriate. Mr P explained:

> You don't ask for people, like, to come round. You don't ask them to like... what do you call them? Relate and that sort of thing, you know — you don't ask for them to come round. You're a bit self-conscious about it all, you know.

> (Interview 12)

In nine interviews, people reported that they did not have particular emotional difficulties. These were not necessarily patients or carers of patients with the best clinical outcomes: one patient was functionally independent, while five were moderately disabled. Five people emphasised that their problems were practical, such as the need to organise adaptations to the house or the desire to move to be closer to family members. Some interviewees who did not report having emotional problems spoke of their resignation to events and ability to 'get on with life,' while others' accounts are marked by self-confidence and 'determination' rather than resignation.

A stroke-specific service?

There were mixed views about the need for a community service for stroke families. Nine people felt that they would have benefited from such a service. Only one of these was functionally independent and, unlike other respondents, she envisaged a service offering face to face counselling:

I'm sure that would have helped me. I just felt as though I'd lost half of my body and nobody seemed to understand. I could have talked to someone on the phone, but it wouldn't have been the same — I really wanted to see someone.

(Interview 5)

Four other carers envisaged a service providing information about what to expect in caring for their relative, reassurance that things were as they should be, and advice on practical issues. Time was also an important factor, with some people highlighting that they would have appreciated, as one person put it, 'time to sit down and discuss with you things you needed to know'.

Three people were equivocal about whether they would have benefited from a community stroke service. They conceded that it may have been useful but the problems they faced had already been resolved by existing services or by virtue of their personal qualities of 'optimism' and 'independence'.

Finally, eight people could see little benefit in the idea. They included four people whose responses emphasised their own ability to cope. Two were patients who were functionally independent and two were carers of people with lower Barthel Index scores. Of the remainder, one respondent did not regard himself as needing any support, since he had accepted the stroke as a consequence of old age and had other, more important concerns. The others were two patients and a carer who all felt that their needs had been adequately met by local health professionals.

Implications for an intervention

Although we have enumerated thematic responses, this study did not aim to quantify levels of need but to explore what problems stroke patients and family members identify and how they would respond to the proposal of a stroke-specific service. A relatively small number of people were interviewed but the sampling strategy aimed to ensure a wide variety of perspectives. Some caution is warranted in interpreting the results because of the length of time after discharge when the interviews were conducted. Had interviews been conducted earlier, more gaps in service provision, for example, may have been identified.

Nevertheless, the qualitative approach allowed people to define their own priorities, identify gaps and preferences for services. As expected, participants identified lack of information and emotional/psychological difficulties in the wake of the stroke. Other issues were also raised: access to on-going physiotherapy or a structured programme of exercises and longer-term monitoring of the patient's progress. The qualitative method also allowed participants to describe their strategies for confronting problems. Thus, there were success stories as well as failures, raising questions about how such successes are achieved. Important elements include individuals' own resources (social, financial, educational, confidence in seeking help) and their expectations about dealing with difficult predicaments and about the roles of family and formal services. Yet the interviews also reveal unevenness in the services actually received from existing providers, including hospital staff and general practice staff.

It also emerged that 'problems' identified by participants may not translate directly into needs with ready solutions. While a clinical need for secondary prevention might be evident to a health professional, avoiding perceived triggers of stress may be more immediately important to the patient who believes that 'stress' causes strokes. Professionals may interpret emotional distress as a need for counselling or other psychological interventions and Stroke Association family support workers prioritise the provision of emotional support (Pound and Wolfe, 1998). While some patients and carers do indeed experience emotional or psychological problems adjusting to the aftermath of stroke, not all regard a professional intervention as necessary, preferring to have information about 'what to expect' or to rely on their own resources. The desire for more therapy may be interpreted by professionals as ignorance of the limitations of functional gains but, to patients themselves, may be related to the maintenance of hope and the desire to continue to be actively working for one's own recovery (Pound *et al*, 1994). Related to this is the desire to have access to on-going monitoring or management.

Conclusion

The study raised a number of questions to consider in developing a new community intervention. First, the unevenness of reported service provision pointed to the need to consider the nature of a community service and how it dovetails with other services. Should it fill in gaps left by other providers, or should it provide a liaison service? As Jolly *et al* (1994) suggested, the effectiveness of liaison services may be limited by the inadequacies of community services currently available and therefore the impact of any coordinating service will depend on the quality of particular services available locally. The diversity of problems people face, the range of resources they bring to a problem and the different expectations they have suggest the need for sensitive targeting of a community service. This should include more than a simple measure of disability, such as the Barthel Index, but should also take into account user identified 'need' and resources. Finally, we should acknowledge that it may not be possible for any one intervention to meet *all* stroke families' needs. Accordingly, any evaluation of such interventions should assess the things the service can realistically hope to influence, rather than the things it cannot.

References

Avis M (1997) Incorporating patients' voices in the audit process. *Qual Health Care* **6**: 86–91

Bisset A, Chesson R (1997) Stroke family care workers. *BMJ* **315**: 606

Crawford M, Rutter D, Manley C, *et al* (2002) Systematic review of involving patients in the planning and development of health care. *BMJ* **325**: 1263

Dennis M, O'Rourke S, Slattery J, Staniforth T, Warlow C (1997) Evaluation of a stroke family care worker: results of a randomised controlled trial. *BMJ* **314**: 1071–7

Dowswell G, Lawler J, Young J, Forster A, Hearn J (1997) A qualitative study of specialist nurse support for stroke patients and care-givers at home. *Clin Rehabil* **11**: 293–30

Fitzpatrick R, Boulton M (1994) Qualitative methods for assessing health care. *Qual Health*

Care **3**: 107–13

Friedland J, McColl M (1992) Social support intervention after stroke: results of a randomized trial. *Arch Phys Med Rehabil* **73**: 573–81

Forster A, Young J (1996) Specialist nurse support for patients with stroke in the community: a randomised controlled trial. *BMJ* **312**: 1642–6

Holbrook M (1982) Stroke: social and emotional outcome. *J R Coll Physicians Lond* **16**: 100–04

Jolly K, Bradley F, Sharp S *et al* (1999) Randomised controlled trial of follow up care in general practice of patients with myocardial infarction and angina: final results of the Southampton heart integrated care project. *BMJ* **318**: 706–11

Lincoln N, Francis V, Lilley S, Sharma J, Summerfield M (2003) Evaluation of a stroke family support organiser: a randomized controlled trial. *Stroke* **34**: 116–21

Mant J, Carter J, Wade D, Winner S (2000) Family support for stroke a randomised controlled trial. *Lancet* **356**: 808–23

Medical Research Council (MRC) (2000) *A Framework for Development and Evaluation of RCTs for Complex Interventions to Improve Health.* MRC, London

McKevitt C, Redfern J, Mold F, Wolfe C (2004) Qualitative studies of stroke: a systematic review. *Stroke* **35**: 1499–505

Pope C, Mays N (1995) Reaching the parts other methods cannot reach: an introduction to qualitative methods in health and health services research. *BMJ* **311**: 42–5

Pound P, Bury M, Gompertz P, Ebrahim S (1994) Views of survivors of stroke on benefits of physiotherapy. *Qual Health Care* **3**: 69–74

Pound P, Gompertz P, Ebrahim S (1997) Study shows importance of patients' feelings. *BMJ* **315**: 606

Pound P, Wolfe C (1998) Support for people living with stroke in the community: the role of the family support organiser. *Br J Ther Rehab* **5**: 482–8

Simpson E, House A (2002) Involving users in the delivery and evaluation of mental health services: systematic review. *BMJ* **325**: 1265

INDEX

non-clinical staff 60, 65
Northern Ireland Chest Heart 74
Nottingham Health Profile 104, 136, 143
Nottingham Stroke Unit 78, 79, 81
nursing staff 78

O

occupational therapists 20, 54, 63, 78, 80, 91, 185
oral hygiene 130
Oxford Community Stroke Project (OCSP) 169

P

Parkinson's disease 114
patient assessment 93
PEG (percutaneous endoscopic gastrostomy feeding) 117–20, 122
perceptual ability 78
perceptual impairment 78
peripheral vascular disease 16
physical disability 101
physiotherapists 63, 66, 85, 88, 90, 93, 95
physiotherapy 19, 85–93, 95–7, 185, 187, 189
Picture Communication Symbols (PCS) 137, 143
pneumonia 128–30
portering 64, 65
Portsmouth Dysphagia Flowcharts (DFC) 126
post-stroke depression (PSD) 99
PowerPoint (Microsoft Office) 65
praxis 18
Present State Examination 102, 106
pressure sores/ulcers 39, 60
primary prevention 71
professional development 70
programme planning 72
PROGRESS (Perindopril Protection against Recurrent Stroke) 7
proprioceptive neuromuscular facilitation 80
psychiatrists 18, 54
psychological problems 9
psychologists 54
pulmonary embolus 5
pulse oximetry 114, 116

Q

quality and audit department 75
quality of life 135–40, 142, 143, 174

R

racism 66
Rapid Estimate of Adult Literacy in Medicine (REALM) 153, 162
Raven's Coloured Progressive Matrices (RCPM) 175, 177
reading 70
recombinant tissue plasminogen activator 6
record keeping 74
recurrence 160
rehabilitation 59–62, 66
renin–angiotensin system 7
resisted exercise 19
risk-factor management 71
Rivermead Mobility Index 88, 96
Rood approach 80
Royal College of Physicians 69, 71, 73, 74, 76
Royal College of Speech and Language Therapists (RCSLT) 126, 130, 150

S

'sick role' 99
safety 20
Safe Implementation of Thrombolysis in Stroke Monitoring Study (SITS-MOST) 15
Scottish Intercollegiate Guidelines Network (SIGN) 135
screening 71
secondary care assessment 71
secondary prevention 16, 21
selective serotonin-reuptake inhibitors (SSRIs) 106
self-confidence 70
self-medication 80
self-neglect 60
sensory impairment 20, 60
service delivery 75
service intervention 86, 96
sexual difficulties 73
Sheffield Screening Test for Acquired Language Disorders (SST) 175
Short Form 36 136
Short Portable Mental Status Questionnaire 173
SMOG readability formula 153
SMOG readability level 151, 159
social isolation 66
social support 22
social worker 53, 54, 70, 72, 74, 183, 185